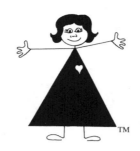

Taking Charge of
FIBROMYALGIA

Fourth Edition

A Self-Management Program
for your
Fibromyalgia Syndrome

Julie Kelly, M.S., R.N.
Rosalie Devonshire, M.S.W.

with contributions by
Jorge Flechas, M.D., M.P.H.
Jenny Fransen, R.N.
Jay A. Goldstein, M.D.
Thomas J. Romano, M.D., Ph.D., FACP, FACR
Jacob Teitelbaum, M.D.

Edited by
Thomas J. Romano, M.D., Ph.D., FACP, FACR

Fibromyalgia Educational Systems, Inc.
500 Bushaway Road • Wayzata, MN 55391-1912
Phone 612/473-6218 • Fax 612/473-6218

NEW JERSEY – Phone 201/785-1128 • Fax 201/785-1129
www.fmsedsys.com

Medical Disclaimer

The treatments and therapies discussed in this handbook are intended for educational purposes only and are not to replace the services of a trained health professional. Consult your physician or health care provider before beginning any medication, treatment or therapy as you may require specific precautions and/or modifications. The authors and editor do not accept liability in the event of negative consequences incurred as a result of information presented in this handbook.

Fibromyalgia Educational Systems, Inc.
500 Bushaway Road • Wayzata, MN 55391-1912
Phone 612/473-6218 • Fax 612/473-6218
NEW JERSEY – Phone 201/785-1128 • Fax 201/785-1129
www.fmsedsys.com

Acknowledgments

Many patients diagnosed with fibromyalgia have limited resources for educating themselves about their condition. We have developed a six-hour self-help class called "Taking Charge of Fibromyalgia," which we have been teaching at Abbott Northwestern Hospital in Minneapolis, Minnesota, since the fall of 1991. The purpose of the class is to educate people with the most up-to-date information on their condition, enabling them to become the primary movers in the management of their fibromyalgia syndrome.

We especially want to recognize Jenny Fransen, R.N., as the originator and contributing author of the "Taking Charge of Fibromyalgia" course. Her vision, contributions and support were critical for the creation of this course and we owe her our deepest thanks.

Many thanks to Donald G. Kocina, who coordinated the production of our most recent edition. We value his expertise and the many contributions he made to this handbook. We also want to thank Lory Strom, who did the word processing for this edition, and Lisa Oelfke, who was responsible for proofreading. Their competence and attention to the details have helped make our handbook what it is today.

This handbook is not designed to take the place of your regular medical doctor's advice. You will want to discuss this information with your doctor and decide with him/her what is appropriate treatment for you.

We have created this handbook and educational program with loving care and dedicate it to all of you who live with this condition. We know how difficult it is and sincerely hope that the future will bring better treatment for all of us. Our deepest thanks to those of you who gave us encouragement to continue with our efforts and to those who provided us with personal experiences of living with fibromyalgia. Your comments were validating and invaluable.

Julie Kelly, M.S., R.N.
Rosalie Devonshire, M.S.W.

About the Authors

Julie Kelly, M.S., R.N., is a fibromyalgia nurse clinician at Abbott Northwestern Hospital in Minneapolis, Minnesota. She works with fibromyalgia patients and their family members in a multi-disciplinary treatment program and educates a variety of health professionals on the diagnosis and treatment of this condition. She co-developed the materials for the *Taking Charge of Fibromyalgia* educational program and is a co-founder of the first fibromyalgia support group in Minnesota. She is married and has two children.

Rosalie Devonshire, M.S.W., is a former teacher, business owner, FMS and CFIDS patient, wife and mother. She works clinically with individuals and families facing non-medical difficulties and provides stress management, biofeedback and psychotherapy treatment to those with physical illnesses. She co-developed the materials for the *Taking Charge of Fibromyalgia* educational program, is co-founder of the first fibromyalgia support group in Minnesota and is a former board member of the Fibromyalgia Alliance of America.

Julie and Rosalie have lectured extensively on the topic of fibromyalgia and bring a personal understanding to their audiences because they too live with fibromyalgia.

Editor

Thomas Romano, M.D., Ph.D., FACP, FACR. We thank him for editing our handbook and offering us advice and guidance.

Contributing Authors

Jorge Flechas, M.D. M.P.H., is a family practitioner in North Carolina who works with many patients who have fibromyalgia (FMS) and patients with chronic fatigue and immune dysfunction syndrome (CFIDS). He has developed a new protocol for treatment of these illnesses using oxytoxin (OT), dehydroepiandrosterone (DHEA) and some natural nutrients. His treatment protocol is discussed in the appendix.

Jenny Fransen, R.N., is a rheumatology nurse clinician and director of the Arthritis Care Program and Fibromyalgia Treatment Program at Abbott Northwestern Hospital in Minneapolis, Minnesota. She is the originator of the *Taking Charge of Fibromyalgia* educational program and co-author of *The Fibromyalgia Help Book.*

Jay Goldstein, M.D., is director of the Chronic Fatigue Syndrome Institute in Anaheim, California. He has treated many CFIDS/FMS patients and has authored a variety of works on these conditions. He is the author of *Chronic Fatigue Syndromes: The Limbic Hypothesis* and *Betrayal by the Brain: The Neurologic Basis of Chronic Fatigue Syndrome, Fibromyalgia Syndrome, and Related Neural Network Disorders.* His protocol is discussed in our section on pioneering treatments and included in the appendix.

Thomas Romano, M.D., Ph.D., FACP, FACR, is a compassionate and dedicated rheumatologist living and practicing in Wheeling, West Virginia. He has treated many FMS patients, authored a number of research articles on the topic and is very interested in the treatment of fibromyalgia. He serves on the Board of Advisors of the American Academy of Pain Management and is on the editorial board of the *Journal of Musculoskeletal Pain.* His treatment protocol for fibromyalgia patients is discussed in the appendix.

Jacob Teitelbaum, M.D., is a board certified physician in internal medicine who practices in Annapolis, Maryland. He has experienced fibromyalgia and chronic fatigue syndrome and also treated patients with these conditions. He is author of *From Fatigued to Fantastic!* An overview of his treatment protocol is discussed in the appendix.

Table of Contents

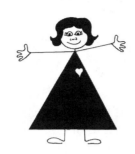

Dear Fibromyalgia

Dear Fibromyalgia,

If you and I are to be constant companions for the rest of my life, I think we should be on speaking terms. First, I must let you know that you will never be able to possess me. You may at times have control of my body, but never my mind or my faith. Also, I am not a quitter. There will always be a battle going on between us. Sometimes you think you are going to win, but it is I who will win the war. For you see, my other companion is God.

Peggy J. Donahue

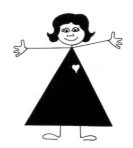

A Fibromyalgia Journal

We feel it is very important to keep a record of your progress for your "Taking Charge of Fibromyalgia" program. Often getting better is a slow and laborious task and it becomes difficult to remember all the details of your program and of your progress. We've designed specific journal pages for this purpose and include one for sleep, medications, coping, exercise, stress management, support and flare-up management. These can be found at the end of the appropriate sections in your handbook. We suggest that you copy these pages, put them in a three-ring binder or folder and start keeping a fibromyalgia journal. Keep your journal in a convenient place and please use it! You will be amazed at how useful it is when you go to your doctor and have an accurate record of your sleep, medications, exercise, etc. (and so will your doctor!). It's also very rewarding to keep track of your progress and to see how much better you're getting. It's the best incentive we know to keep up with all the components of your "Taking Charge of Fibromyalgia" program. It may be helpful to delegate some pages in your journal for "worry time," those 10 to 20 minutes a day when you write down all your worries. You might even sleep better!

Make your journal work for you. It can be an important component of taking charge of your fibromyalgia.

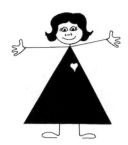

History of Fibromyalgia

Jenny Fransen, R.N.

Muscular rheumatism was first described over 150 years ago. In fact, some believe that even the biblical sufferings of Job were those of a fibromyalgia patient: "The night racks my bones, and the pain that gnaws me takes no rest" (Job 30:17). In 1904, Gowers first used the term "fibrositis" to describe the muscle pain syndrome that we know today as fibromyalgia. The term "fibrositis" was used to describe what was believed at that time to be an inflammation of the soft tissue and muscular fibrous tissue.

During the 1950s and 1960s, fibrositis was considered to have a psychological origin. Since that time, research has been inconclusive in proving that inflammation or abnormality of the muscle tissue exists. For that reason the term "fibrositis" does not accurately describe the condition.

Travell defined myofascial pain syndrome as a condition of tenderness and pain in the muscles that is related to trigger points, which are sometimes associated with a taut muscle band that can be palpated, or felt, with the hand. Trigger points are defined as tenderness or pain in the muscle that usually causes referred pain. Referred pain is pain or deep aching that is made worse by palpating this abnormality in the muscle, the taut band, which spreads or radiates beyond the muscle area that is palpated. Myofascial pain syndrome is usually limited to a certain group or several groups of muscles. Fibromyalgia commonly can create muscle pain that is more widespread, affecting more of the body, as well as having more of a chronic nature.

There has been confusion between the two conditions of fibromyalgia and myofascial pain syndrome, and often the terms trigger point and tender point are used interchangeably even though they may not be the same.

In the 1970s, Smythe began defining the problem as widespread pain and aching with local tenderness, accompanying fatigue, morning stiffness, and a worsening of pain with activity. He began to propose its underlying causes, as well as standardized criteria to diagnose patients with fibromyalgia.

Later, during the 1970s, rheumatologists began to develop the diagnostic criteria, or standard set of symptoms that must be met in order for the diagnosis to be made.

In 1981, Yunus and Katz renamed it "fibromyalgia" or fibromyalgia syndrome, since a number of symptoms other than muscle pain and tenderness were found to exist together as a syndrome. Yunus was responsible for further defining the symptoms and tender points. It was during this period that the foundation of today's comprehensive treatment approach was begun, which utilizes different types of treatments and therapies together to bring about an improvement in symptoms.

Kellgren observed that in fibromyalgia, the pain came from deep below the surface of the muscle. His research showed that there was irritation of fascia, tendon, and muscle producing pain that radiated, leading to more research that gave us information on trigger points and trigger areas.

Smythe defined the problem as widespread pain and aching with local tenderness with accompanying fatigue, morning stiffness, and a worsening of pain with activity, without apparent cause. He offered a hypothesis to the cause of this condition, as well as criteria to help with more accurate diagnoses.

Over the past decade we have had an explosion of research into the pathogenesis, or origin, of fibromyalgia. Yet there remains much to be learned.

REFERENCES

Reilly, P., Littlejohn, G. History of Fibromyalgia. *Journal of Musculoskeletal Pain*, 1(2), 1993.

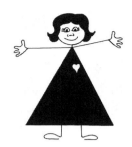

Diagnosis and Symptoms

Fibromyalgia syndrome (FMS) is characterized by widespread musculoskeletal pain, aching and stiffness with associated sleep disturbances and fatigue. It is seen in all age groups from young children to the elderly, with many patients experiencing their initial symptoms in their 20s and 30s. The majority of adult patients are women, experiencing this condition seven to eight times more often than men. In school age children, boys and girls are affected about equally. The symptoms and treatment are generally the same among men, women and children.

The prevalence of fibromyalgia syndrome in the general population was studied by Fred Wolfe, M.D., and found to be approximately 2%. Other findings by Wolfe, et al., were 3.4% of women and 0.5% of men in the communities studied met the American College of Rheumatology criteria for the diagnosis of fibromyalgia. Similar prevalence rates have been found worldwide.

Among individuals with fibromyalgia syndrome, there is a variable onset of symptoms. Some individuals recall a specific triggering event associated with an abrupt onset of symptoms. The triggering event could be

▲ **Physical trauma**
▲ **Emotional trauma**
▲ **Flu or other viral illness**
▲ **Nonviral infection**

▲ **Sudden hormonal change**
▲ **Steroid withdrawal**
▲ **Hypothyroidism**
▲ **Extended disruption of sleep**

Some individuals report that their symptoms began for no obvious reason. Others describe a very gradual onset of their symptoms over many years.

Some individuals experience musculoskeletal pain and tender points only in one particular region of their body and may have what some researchers call "regional fibromyalgia (RF)." A subgroup of these individuals report that over time, their pain "grows" to gradually affect many areas of their body, developing the widespread pain of fibromyalgia syndrome (FMS). In a recent study of regional fibromyalgia patients by Yunus, et al., a majority of RF patients felt better after a mean follow-up period of 5.8 years, but about 40% developed widespread pain. This finding suggests an overlap between regional fibromyalgia and fibromyalgia syndrome.

The course of fibromyalgia for many is characterized by periods of remission and flare-ups which vary in length and severity. It is a condition that is invisible to others and is not life threatening. Many individuals with FMS learn to manage their symptoms quite well, especially after learning about FMS and actively participating in the appropriate treatment. Unfortunately there are some who experience more persistent symptoms. These individuals may have another illness and/or injury which contributes to the complexity of their treatment, making management of their symptoms more difficult.

The diagnosis of fibromyalgia is made from your history and a detailed musculoskeletal exam. The absence of certain symptoms and signs is just as important as the presence of certain characteristics.

Positive and Negative Diagnostic Features of Fibromyalgia

	Positive	*Negative*
History	Patient complains of chronic diffuse pain, paresthesias	Normal history in respects other than pain, e.g., no joint swelling, no redness
Constitutional symptoms	Fatigue, sleep disturbance	No fever or major weight loss
Joint examination	Pain on full motion may be present	No joint effusions or deformities
Muscle examination	Tenderness at certain muscle-tendon junctions and muscle bellies, muscle tightness	No muscle weakness or atrophy
Neurologic examination	No characteristic positive findings	No sensory or motor abnormalities
Laboratory studies	No characteristic positive findings with routine testing	Normal complete blood count, erythrocyte sedimentation rate, muscle enzymes, thyroid function

Goldenberg, D. L., M.D. Diagnostic and therapeutic challenges of fibromyalgia. *Hospital Practice*, 1989, September 30.

The American College of Rheumatology 1990 Criteria for the Classification of Fibromyalgia*

▲ History of widespread pain for at least 3 months

Definition. Pain is considered widespread when all of the following are present: pain on the left side of the body, pain on the right side of the body, pain above the waist, and pain below the waist. In addition, axial skeletal pain (cervical spine or anterior chest or thoracic spine or low back) must be present. In this definition, shoulder and buttock pain is considered as pain for each involved side. "Low back" pain is considered lower segment pain.

▲ Pain in 11 of 18 tender point sites on digital palpation

Definition. Pain, on digital palpation, must be present in at least 11 of the following 18 tender point sites:

Occiput: bilateral, at the suboccipital muscle insertions.

Low cervical: bilateral, at the anterior aspects of the intertransverse spaces at C5-C7.

Trapezius: bilateral, at the midpoint of the upper border.

Supraspinatus: bilateral, at origins, above the scapula spine near the medial border.

Second rib: bilateral, at the second costochondral junctions, just lateral to the junctions on upper surfaces.

Lateral epicondyle: bilateral, 2 cm distal to the epicondyles.

Gluteal: bilateral, in upper outer quadrants of buttocks in anterior fold of muscle.

Greater trochanter: bilateral, posterior to the trochanteric prominence.

Knee: bilateral, at the medial fat pad proximal to the joint line.

Illustration of Tender Points

Arthritis Foundation, Atlanta, Georgia, 30326.
Fibromyalgia (Fibrositis), 1992.

Digital palpation should be performed with an approximate force of 4 kg.

For a tender point to be considered "positive," the subject must state that the palpation was painful. "Tender" is not to be considered "painful."

---

* For classification purposes, patients will be said to have fibromyalgia if both criteria are satisfied. Widespread pain must have been present for at least three months. The presence of a second clinical disorder does not exclude the diagnosis of fibromyalgia. The American College of Rheumatology. Criteria for the classification of fibromyalgia. *Arthritis and Rheumatism*, 33 (2), 1990, February.

DIAGNOSIS

Symptoms of Fibromyalgia Syndrome

There are a number of symptoms associated with fibromyalgia syndrome. You may or may not experience all of the symptoms listed below, but will likely experience the more common symptoms of

- ▲ **Muscle pain**
- ▲ **Tender points**
- ▲ **Sleep disturbance**

Other symptoms associated with FMS are

- ▲ **Fatigue**
- ▲ **Subjective swelling**
- ▲ **Joint pain**
- ▲ **Neurological symptoms**
- ▲ **Headache**

- ▲ **Irritable bowel syndrome**
- ▲ **Irritable bladder**
- ▲ **Morning stiffness**
- ▲ **Raynaud's phenomenon**
- ▲ **Memory problems**

Symptoms of fibromyalgia vary considerably among people.

Additional Reported Symptoms

In recent years, a number of research findings have broadened the understanding of fibromyalgia and have included a greater array of symptoms now thought to be associated with this condition. Research suggests that individuals with FMS are not just tender in specific tender point areas, but are more sensitive to painful stimuli throughout the body. The comment that "I hurt all over" certainly makes sense when viewed in this context.

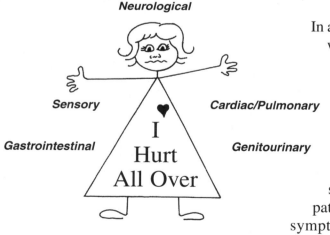

In a 1992 study of 554 individuals with FMS compared with a group of 169 controls, Waylonis and Heck also reported a number of additional symptoms that appeared to be associated with fibromyalgia. "Individuals with fibromyalgia self report a greater incidence of bursitis, chondromalacia, constipation, diarrhea, temporomandibular joint dysfunction, vertigo, sinus and thyroid problems. Symptomatic complaints found statistically more prevalent in fibromyalgia patients, included concentration problems, sensory symptoms, swollen glands and tinnitus. Other associations occurring with significant increased frequency were chronic cough, coccygeal and pelvic pain, tachycardia and weakness." Twelve percent of the participants reported that they had children with symptoms of fibromyalgia and 25% reported that they had symptomatic parents. Of the participants, 70% noted that their symptoms were aggravated by noise, lights, stress, posture and weather.

The following table by Daniel Clauw, M.D., illustrates the wide variety of additional symptoms and syndromes now linked to fibromyalgia.

Symptoms & Syndromes
Now Linked to Fibromyalgia

Neurological
- Paresthesia: numbness or tingling (non-dermatomal).
- Headaches: tension and migraine.
- Neurogenic inflammation: inflammatory sensation (rashes, itching, inflammation) initiated by nerves. A discrete, localized inflammatory response which does not activate the immune system or show up on tests.
- Cognitive: difficulty with concentration and short-term memory.

Sensory
- Auditory: low frequency, sensorineural hearing loss; decreased painful sound threshold.[1]
- Vestibular: exaggerated nystagmus (involuntary rapid movement of the eyeball), dizziness, vertigo.[1]
- Ocular: impaired function of smooth muscles used for focus as well as skeletal muscles used for tracking.[2]

Cardiac Pulmonary
- Mitral valve prolapse–a benign cardiac condition; 75% incidence in fibromyalgia patients according to one study.[3] Disorder may be due to neurological hyperactivity rather than a defect in the heart valve.
- Heart palpitations.
- Non-cardiac chest pain which may simulate cardiac disorder.
- Abnormal smooth muscle tone in muscles surrounding the bronchi of the lungs.[4]

Gastrointestinal[5]
- Heartburn.
- Irritable bowel syndrome.
- Esophageal dysmotility: objective abnormalities in smooth muscle functioning and tone in the esophagus; 40-70% incidence according to one study.

Genitourinary
- Painful menstruation.
- Increased urinary frequency and urgency.[6]
- Increased incidence of interstitial cystitis.[7]
- Vulvar vestibulitis or vulvodynia: characterized by a painful vulvar region and painful sexual intercourse.[8]

Miscellaneous
- Joint hypermobility.
- Temporomandibular joint disorder: in many fibromyalgia patients, problems are encountered because of the abnormal tone in muscles around the joint–not because of abnormalities in the joint itself.
- Plantar arch or heel pain.

References

(1) Gerster, J. and A. HadjDjilani, Hearing and Vestibular Abnormalities in Primary Fibrositis Syndrome. *J. Rheumatol*, 1984. 11: p. 678-80.

(2) Rosenhall, U., G. Johansson, and G. Orndahl, Eye Motility Dysfunction In Primary Fibromyalgia With Dysesthesia. *Scand J Rehab Med*, 1987. 19: p. 139-45.

(3) Pellegrino, M., D. Van Fossen, C. Gordon, J. Ryan, G. Waylonis, Prevalence Of Mitral Valve Prolapse In Primary Fibromyalgia: A Pilot Investigation. *Arch Phys Med Rehabil*, 1989. 70: p. 541-3.

(4) Lurie, M., K. Caidahl, G. Johansson, B. Bake, Respiratory Function In Chronic Primary Fibromyalgia. *Scand J. Rehabil Med*, 1990. 22: p. 151-5.

(5) Hiltz, R., P. Gupta, K. Maher, et al., Low Threshold Of Visceral Nociception And Significant Upper Gastrointestinal Pathology In Patients With Fibromyalgia Syndrome. *Arthritis Rheum*, 1993. 36(9S): p. C93.

(6) Wallace, D., Genitourinary Manifestations Of Fibrositis: An Increased Association With The Female Urethral Syndrome. *J. Rheumatol*, 1990. 17: p. 238-9.

(7) Koziol, J., D. Clark, R. Gittes, E. Tan, The Natural History Of Interstitial Cystitis. *J. Urology*, 1993. 149: p. 465-9.

(8) Friedrich, E., Vulvar Vestibulitis Syndrome. *J Reproduct Med*, 1987. 32(2): p. 110-4.

(9) Cleveland, C. Jr., R. Fisher, E. Brestel, J. Esinhart, W. Metzger, Chronic Rhinitis: An Under-recognized Association With Fibromyalgia. *Allergy Proc*, 1992. 13: p. 263-7.

DIAGNOSIS

Table and references are printed with permission from an article entitled "New Insights into Fibromyalgia" by Daniel Clauw, M.D. Article was published in *Fibromyalgia Frontiers*, 2(4), Fall 1994.

Modulating Factors

Modulating factors are those which influence the symptoms of your fibromyalgia. Some modulating factors are as follows:

- ▲ **Lack of or too much physical activity**
- ▲ **Weather changes**
- ▲ **Depression**
- ▲ **Major stressful events**
- ▲ **PMS**

- ▲ **Postural strain**
- ▲ **Anxiety**
- ▲ **Repetitive and mechanical stress**
- ▲ **Interrupted sleep**
- ▲ **Illness**

Fibromyalgia in Children

Juvenile primary fibromyalgia syndrome (JPFS) is a common but often overlooked rheumatologic condition. It is known to affect school age boys and girls about equally. The symptoms are comparable with those in adults with fibromyalgia. In a study by T. J. Romano, M.D., all of the children reported diffuse musculoskeletal pain. Stiffness was present in 67% of the children and 33% had complaints of soft tissue swelling. Other frequent symptoms that were reported were fatigue (100%), poor sleep/waking up tired (73%) and headaches (53%). An examination revealed typical tender points, no joint swelling, nodules or fluid in a joint and an absence of neurological findings. Standard laboratory tests were normal. Similar results were found in studies by Yunus and Masi and by Calabro. The most common aggravating factors were cold and/or humid weather, physical overactivity or inactivity, anxiety/stress and poor sleep. The treatment for children with fibromyalgia is generally the same as with adults.

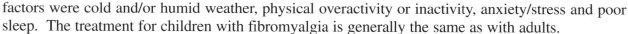

If you suspect that your child may have juvenile primary fibromyalgia syndrome, it's important to have him/her evaluated by a physician who is very familiar with this condition. (Many pediatricians are not familiar with JPFS.) Unfortunately, though fibromyalgia is common in children, it is frequently confused with other conditions, especially juvenile rheumatoid arthritis. In order to avoid unwarranted testing and investigation and possibly improper management, it is important to have JPFS correctly diagnosed as soon as possible. Education of both the parents and child should then follow the diagnosis. This educational process is often very helpful in allaying many of the fears of both parent and child. It also elicits their participation in the subsequent treatment program.

An excellent resource for parents and their children is *Fibromyalgia Syndrome and Chronic Fatigue Syndrome in Young People,* edited by Kristin Thorson (1994). Copies of this booklet may be obtained from Fibromyalgia Network, P.O. Box 3175, Tucson, AZ 85751-1750. (800) 853-2929, fax (520) 290-5550. The cost is $10.00 in U.S. and Canada.

Primary Fibromyalgia Syndrome and Chronic Fatigue Syndrome

Are primary fibromyalgia syndrome and chronic fatigue syndrome the same condition? The many similarities between FMS and CFIDS have presented researchers with the challenge to continue to reassess the criteria for diagnosing both syndromes.

During the 1980s, Don Goldenberg, M.D., and Anthony Komaroff, M.D., showed that there were no significant differences between FMS and CFIDS when symptoms, tender points and demographics were assessed. In fact, 75% of the patients diagnosed with CFIDS also met the tender point criteria for FMS. Many patients diagnosed with fibromyalgia syndrome could also have been diagnosed as having chronic fatigue syndrome. H. Moldofsky, M.D., has discussed that no differences were found between these two patient groups in several other studies when brain function, sleep physiology and immunology were compared.

Do CFIDS and FMS anchor the opposite ends of a continuum of symptoms, with those patients diagnosed with CFIDS presenting with a primary symptom of overwhelming fatigue and those patients diagnosed with FMS presenting with a primary symptom of aches and pains? There seems to be little disagreement among many physicians that CFIDS and FMS at the very least share many common symptoms and that their treatment is very similar. Would one's diagnosis of CFIDS or FMS be different depending on which specialist initially assessed the patient?

The following is a case definition for chronic fatigue syndrome (CFIDS) as published in the December 1994 *Annals of Internal Medicine.*

Chronic Fatigue Syndrome

Fatigue:
Patients must have otherwise unexplained, relapsing fatigue that is new (not life-long); not the result of ongoing exertion; not relieved by rest; and that results in substantial decrease in levels of occupational, social, educational, or personal activities.

Symptoms:
The patient must have four or more of the following eight symptoms. Symptoms must persist for six months and the patient must not have predated fatigue.

▲ **Self-reported impairment of memory or concentration that affects occupational, social, educational, or personal activities**

▲ **Sore throat**

▲ **Tender cervical (neck area) or axillary (underarm area) nodes**

▲ **Myalgias (muscle pain)**

▲ **Arthralgias (pain along the nerve of a joint) – no redness or swelling**

▲ **Headache of a new type**

▲ **Unrefreshing sleep**

▲ **Post-exertional malaise, lasting at least 24 hours**

If you have chronic sore throats, low-grade fevers of unknown origin and/or chronic colds, you may want to discuss these symptoms with your physician to rule out an Epstein Barr viral infection, cytomegaloviral infection, HMV 6 or other infectious agents. Depending on your test results, other types of treatment may be appropriate.

The FMS/CFIDS controversy continues to intrigue researchers and will no doubt be further studied and investigated. While we, as patients, watch with interest for new studies on this subject to be published, we will best spend our energy on treating our symptoms and focusing on getting better. Let's leave this controversy to the researchers!

▲▲▲

Diagnosis and Symptoms

▲ Be sure that the physician who diagnosed you with fibromyalgia did a tender point exam. If he/she did not, ask him/her to do one. This is an important diagnostic tool. A 15-minute video that illustrates the correct methods of performing the tender point exam is available. Ordering information is noted in the resource section.

▲ If you are seeing a physician or other healthcare professional who is not familiar with fibromyalgia, either provide him or her with some educational materials on fibromyalgia or seek out someone familiar with this condition.

REFERENCES

Arthritis Foundation, Atlanta, Georgia, 30326. *Fibromyalgia (Fibrositis)*, 1992.

Bonafide, R.P., Downey, D.C., Bennett, R.M. An association of fibromyalgia with primary Sjogren's syndrome: a prospective study of 72 patients. *Journal of Rheumatology*, 22(1), 133-136, January 1995.

Buchwald, D., Garrity, D. Comparison of patients with chronic fatigue syndrome, fibromyalgia, and multiple chemical sensitivities. *Arch Intern. Med.*, 154(18), 2049-53, September 26, 1994.

Calabro, J. Fibromyalgia (Fibrositis) in children. *The American Journal of Medicine*, 81 (Suppl. 3A), 1986, September 29.

Clauw, D. New insights into fibromyalgia. *Fibromyalgia Frontiers*, 2(4), Fall 1994.

Goldenberg, D.L., et al. High frequency of fibromyalgia in patients with chronic fatigue seen in a primary care practice. *Arthritis Rheum*, 33(3), 381-387, 1990.

Goldenberg, D.L., Diagnostic and therapeutic challenges of fibromyalgia. *Hospital Practice*, 1989, September 30.

Krilou, L. Chronic fatigue syndrome. *Pediatric Annals*, 24(6), 290-294, June 1995.

Moldofsky, H. Nonrestorative sleep and symptoms after a febrile illness in patients with FMS and CFIDS. *Journal of Rheumatology*, 16(Suppl 19), 150-153, 1989.

Nishikai, Nasahiko. Primary fibromyalgia and chronic fatigue syndrome: are these diseases identical? *Journal of Musculoskeletal Pain*, 3(1), 40, 1995.

Reid, G.J., Lang, B.A., and McGrath, P.J. Primary juvenile fibromyalgia: psychological adjustment, family functioning, coping and functional disability. *Arthritis and Rheumatism*, 40(1), 752-760, 1997.

Romano, T.J. Fibromyalgia in children; diagnosis and treatment. *The West Virginia Medical Journal*, 87, 1991, March.

The American College of Rheumatology. Criteria for the classification of fibromyalgia. *Arthritis and Rheumatism*, 33 (2), 1990, February.

Waylonis, G.W., and Heck, W. Fibromyalgia syndrome. *American Journal of Physical Medicine and Rehabilitation*, 71 (6), 1992, December.

Wolfe, F., Ross, K., Anderson, J., Russell, I.J., and Hebert. L. The prevalence and characteristics of fibromyalgia in the general population. *Arthritis Rheum*, 38(1), 19-28, 1995.

Yunus, M.B., and Masi, A.T. Juvenile primary fibromyalgia syndrome: a clinical study of thirty three patients and matched controls. *Arthritis and Rheumatism*, 28, 1985.

Yunus, M.B., del Castillo, L.D., and Aldaq, J.C. Prognosis of regional fibromyalgia (RF). University of Illinois College of Medicine, Peoria, IL 61605. Poster session at 1994 ACR/ARHP Annual Meeting, October, 1994.

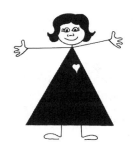

Medical Conditions Commonly Occurring Together with Fibromyalgia

- ▲ Lyme disease
- ▲ Post-polio syndrome
- ▲ HIV infections
- ▲ Rheumatoid arthritis
- ▲ Osteoarthritis
- ▲ Polymyalgia rheumatica
- ▲ Cancer
- ▲ Ankylosing spondylitis
- ▲ Hypothyroidism

- ▲ Endometriosis
- ▲ PMS
- ▲ TMJ dysfunction
- ▲ Cervical and lumbar disc disease
- ▲ Connective tissue diseases
- ▲ Myofascial pain
- ▲ Neurologic disorders
- ▲ Chronic fatigue syndrome
- ▲ Sjogren's syndrome

Many doctors are now diagnosing fibromyalgia more readily and occasionally may miss other medical conditions which are frequently present along with fibromyalgia.

Make sure your doctor checks you for any of these conditions which could mimic fibromyalgia symptoms or are often found along with fibromyalgia. If you have any of these or any other illness, you'll want that treated, as any illness may make your FMS symptoms worse.

Lyme disease: Following a deer tick bite a person can develop fibromyalgia-like symptoms with the exception of inflamed joints and a fever. Although there is a blood test for lyme disease, it is not always conclusive, so a doctor must diagnose it using his or her clinical judgment. Antibiotics are used in its treatment and will not be effective for fibromyalgia symptoms. Many lyme patients can develop fibromyalgia.

Post-polio syndrome: Muscle weakness rather than pain occurs. A blood test usually shows elevated serum muscle enzyme levels.

HIV Infections: About one-third of HIV patients develop fibromyalgia. A blood test shows if you are HIV positive.

Rheumatoid arthritis: Generalized stiffness and aching, symptoms usually restricted to joints, not muscles, with swelling, warmth and tenderness. A blood test is usually positive for rheumatoid factor.

Osteoarthritis: Presents similarly to fibromyalgia; patient will not have tender points. X-rays show degenerative changes of bones.

Polymyalgia rheumatica: A blood test confirms this disease, usually found in people over age 50. Patients respond well to cortisone.

Cancer: Many cancers can cause pain and fatigue and in certain circumstances appropriate measures to rule out cancer should be considered. Many cancer patients develop fibromyalgia during the course of their cancer.

Ankylosing spondylitis: X-rays show changes in the spine and there is limited motion of the spine. There is no cure and it is treated with NSAIDs.

Hypothyroidism: Can cause symptoms that mimic fibromyalgia. A blood test will confirm the diagnosis.

Endometriosis: Many patients with endometriosis develop fibromyalgia.

PMS: Fibromyalgia symptoms are sometimes worse during this phase of the menstrual cycle.

TMJ dysfunction: Many fibromyalgia patients have TMJ dysfunction characterized by locking or clicking of the jaw with associated pain. Your dentist can evaluate this condition and recommend treatment.

Cervical and lumbar disc disease: Can cause pain and can be diagnosed by your doctor and with x-rays.

Connective tissue diseases: These include lupus and Sjogren's syndrome. This is diagnosed with a blood test, although about 10% of healthy women have a low positive result for this blood test. False positives can also occur in the elderly.

Myofascial pain: Pain of unknown origin usually localized to one area of the body rather than all over as in fibromyalgia; no fatigue is associated with it.

Neurologic disorders: Multiple sclerosis or Parkinson's Disease can cause neurologic symptoms such as numbness or tingling, burning and fatigue. Neurologic tests such as an EMG and nerve conduction studies can rule out a neurologic disorder.

Chronic fatigue syndrome (CFIDS): Many doctors think CFIDS and fibromyalgia are the same entity; some think they are different. There seems to be little disagreement that CFIDS and FMS at the very least share many common symptoms and that their treatment is very similar among many physicians. An infectious disease doctor is a specialist who often treats CFIDS.

Sjogren's syndrome: A chronic inflammatory and autoimmune disorder characterized by diminished tears and saliva (dry eyes and mouth).

If you have any of these conditions, your fibromyalgia symptoms could be exacerbated, so it is important to have them properly diagnosed and treated.

REFERENCES

Bennett, R.M., Smythe, H.A., Wolfe. Recognizing fibromyalgia. *Patient Care,* 23: 60-83, July 15, 1989.

Schumacher, R. *Primer on the Rheumatic Diseases.* 9th edition, Atlanta: Arthritis Foundation, 1988.

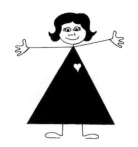

Research

Putting the Pieces Together

We believe it is important to cover the research aspect of FMS in this handbook and our seminar, because so many patients have been told their symptoms are all in their heads. Some have also been told that if they would learn to relax and get rid of the stress in their lives, the symptoms of FMS would go away. This has not proven to be the case, and we want you, the FMS patient, to know and be assured that there really is something going on physically in your body. We have tried to make this as easy to understand as possible, without leaving out important data. Kristin Thorson, editor of the *Fibromyalgia Network,* does an excellent job of keeping subscribers informed of new developments in research, treatments, and medications. Ordering information for this newsletter and other excellent publications is listed in the resource section for your convenience. We feel an educated patient is one who will receive quality treatment from his/her medical team and has the best chance of coping effectively with this condition. Other FMS organizations are listed as resources at the end of the book for you to use as well. Please avail yourself of these resources and keep current with advances in research and treatment. You wouldn't want to miss out on any medical discovery which might help you feel better!

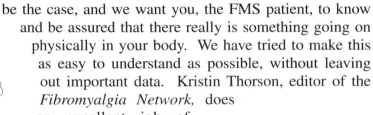

Researchers Are Searching for the Key Which Will Unlock the FMS Puzzle

Areas of Research

- ▲ Psychological states
- ▲ Central nervous system
- ▲ Adrenal-pituitary-hypothalamus-thyroid-axis
- ▲ Muscle abnormalities

- ▲ Amino acids
- ▲ Magnesium
- ▲ Brain scans
- ▲ Immune system
- ▲ Limbic system
- ▲ Genetic studies

Abnormalities in Many Systems:
FMS Is a Physical Problem

At this time, no single mechanism has been discovered as the cause of FMS. Researchers have found abnormalities in various systems in the body, but have not been able to tie these together. Much progress has been made in recent years, as more researchers have become interested in FMS and as more funds have become available.

Is This All in Your Head?
Definitely Not!

Many researchers have been searching for a psychological cause for the symptoms of FMS. The studies done in this area are conflicting, as some studies have shown a high incidence of depression in FMS patients, while others show a normal prevalence. Robert Bennett, M.D., is just one of the many physicians who now feel that the depression patients experience is often due to the pain, fatigue, and stresses of living with an illness that can cause so much disability. The fact that the treatment options are so inadequate can contribute to an anxious, irritable and depressed patient. It is well known that many chronically ill patients with rheumatoid arthritis, cancer, lupus, etc., develop depression as the result of living with their illness. The FMS patient is no exception. We want you to understand that you are not the cause of your illness, nor are you the cause of your depression. It is very important to have your depression treated if you do become depressed, because it can aggravate your FMS symptoms.

Central Nervous System Dysfunction

Controls:

- ▲ Sleep
- ▲ Pain
- ▲ Mood
- ▲ Hunger

- ▲ Memory
- ▲ Emotions
- ▲ Thirst
- ▲ Muscle movement

Central Nervous System Could Be Hyperactive

Sensitive to:

- ▲ Bright lights
- ▲ Loud noises
- ▲ Smells

- ▲ Chemicals
- ▲ Foods
- ▲ Drugs

Robert Bennett, M.D., and I. Jon Russell, M.D., believe that at this time evidence is pointing to a central nervous system dysfunction in the pathology of FMS. The central nervous system is one of the two main divisions of the nervous system of the body. Through messages sent by chemicals the body manufactures, the central nervous system controls sleep, pain, mood, muscle movement, hunger and many other functions. It

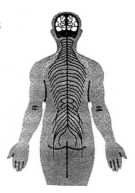

is made up of the brain and spinal cord and is the main network of coordination and control for the entire body. Daniel Clauw, M.D., feels that FMS patients' central nervous systems are hyperactive and overly responsive to stimuli from the environment. This could be why so many patients are sensitive to bright lights, loud noises, noxious smells, drugs, and pain.

Neurotransmitters
Chemical Link between Brain and Rest of the Body

Neurotransmitters are chemicals released from nerve endings which transmit impulses across the gaps between the nerves and the muscles or glands that the nerves supply. The neurotransmitters function as the chemical link between your brain and the rest of your body. Through messages sent by the neurotransmitters, the central nervous system controls sleep, pain, mood, muscle movement, hunger and many other important functions. When the levels of these chemicals are abnormal in the body, they can create havoc.

↓ Serotonin ↓

- ▲ Depression
- ▲ Anxiety
- ▲ Pain
- ▲ Immune system
- ▲ Sleep
- ▲ Smooth muscle function

Serotonin, one neurotransmitter, was found in low levels in some FMS patients by I. Jon Russell, M.D. Serotonin helps to control depression, anxiety, pain levels, immune system function, vascular (blood vessel) constriction/dilation, smooth muscle function, sleep and many other functions.

↑ Substance P ↑
Switched on Nerve Endings
! Pain!

Substance P is another neurotransmitter which was found to be three times higher in FMS patients' spinal fluid by Dr. Russell and also by Dr. Henning Vaeroy. This neurotransmitter is responsible for pain transmission. It is theorized that when serotonin is low and substance P is high, we feel more pain.

When serotonin is low and substance P is high, pain is high.

Low Levels of Many Neurochemicals

- ▲ Catecholamines
- ▲ Norepinephrine
- ▲ Epinephrine
- ▲ Dopamine
- ▲ Growth hormone
- ▲ Thytropin-releasing hormone
- ▲ Cortisol
- ▲ DHEAS

Other neurotransmitters, called catecholamines, were also found in low concentrations in the spinal fluid by Dr. Russell. These are the metabolite products (substance produced during metabolism) of norepinephrine, epinephrine, and dopamine. These chemicals are needed for various processes in the body, but their main job is to prepare the body to act in times of stress—which is called the "fight or flight syndrome" and includes increased blood pressure, faster heart rate, and faster breathing.

Serotonin, norepinephrine, and dopamine stimulate growth hormone which has also been found in low amounts in some FMS patients. Growth hormone is needed for normal muscle metabolism and repair, and 80% of it is secreted by the pituitary gland during deep level sleep. Could our disturbed sleep cycles have something to do with growth hormone or vice-versa? Robert Bennett, M.D., has been researching this aspect of FMS and has finished a study on supplementing FMS patients with growth hormone. Though it did prove effective in relieving some symptoms of FMS, growth hormone is an expensive treatment at this time and is not readily available for general treatment of FMS.

This Is a Complex Network which Interacts Closely—Seems to Be Dysregulated

▲ **Hypothalamus**   ▲ **Thyroid**
▲ **Pituitary gland**   ▲ **Brain**
▲ **Adrenals**   ▲ **Central nervous system**

The hypothalamus, pituitary, adrenals, thyroid, brain and central nervous system are part of a complex network in which all work closely together. It seems that many chemicals involved with these systems are low in FMS patients. The thyroid is a gland which secretes another hormone that is responsible for energy levels, metabolic rate, body temperature, regulation of protein, fat, and carbohydrate processing in all cells, growth hormone release, central nervous system growth, stimulation of the making of many enzymes and is needed for muscle tone. The thyroid is activated by the pituitary gland. Although many FMS patients' thyroid tests are normal, Dr. Russell states that about one-third of FMS patients develop a thyroid disorder such as hypothyroidism, which occurs when the thyroid gland does not receive enough thyroid stimulating hormone from the pituitary and cannot produce enough thyroid hormones. When this happens, weight gain, muscle pain, dry/itchy skin, constipation, and cold sensitivity can occur.

In two separate studies by Ferraccioli and Neeck, FMS patients were found to have a low response to thytropin-releasing hormone, which is released by the hypothalamus and causes the pituitary to secrete thyroid stimulating hormone (TSH). It does seem as if there is a problem with the hypothalamus, pituitary and the thyroid, and further research needs to be carried out to establish definitive answers. If you find your thyroid level is low (determined by a blood test performed by a doctor), you will need to take a thyroid hormone which must be monitored closely because too much can cause nervousness, rapid heart rate, and other abnormalities. Thyroid hormone supplements may not take away all of your FMS symptoms, but could help increase your energy level or reduce your pain.

Nerve growth factor, a protein necessary for the repair of certain neurons which help to trigger release of substance P, was found elevated in FMS patients. Researchers need to find out the reason for this and also why another neurotransmitter called neuropeptide Y (thought to be a long-acting, more stable form of norepinephrine) was found in lower levels in FMS/CFIDS patients.

In another study, Glenn McCain, M.D., found low cortisol levels in FMS patients. Cortisol is a steroid hormone found naturally in the body which helps reduce swelling. The adrenal gland secretes cortisol as well as another chemical called DHEAS (dehydroepiandrosterone-sulfate), which was found in lower than normal concentrations by I. Jon Russell, M.D. DHEAS is the first metabolite of DHEA, a steroid-like hormone involved in cellular growth and development. It naturally decreases with the aging process. Low DHEAS levels corresponded with high pain levels in this study. A few doctors are now prescribing DHEA for their patients, and some patients are reporting that they are experiencing an improved sense of well-being, more energy, and less pain from DHEA supplements. Suggested doses are 5 to 60 mg. You could talk with your physician about DHEA, as there have been no studies published on it yet. DHEA is now available in health food stores, without a prescription, although potency cannot be guaranteed.

Muscle Abnormalities
Is There Something Wrong with FMS Patients' Muscles?

▲ **No inflammation**
▲ **Uneven distribution of oxygen**
▲ **Low levels of ATP, ADP and phosphocreatine**
▲ **Low aerobic capability**
▲ **Erratic breathing pattern**
▲ **Low exercising blood flow**
▲ **Reduced grip strength**
▲ **Heightened response to muscle microtrauma**
▲ **Low levels of a substance which helps repair muscle tissue**
▲ **Found phosphodiester peaks—normally appears in elderly**

FMS abnormalities are not only in the muscles but are also in the central nervous system

For many years, researchers thought the problem of FMS was in the muscles themselves. This would make sense, since this is where FMS sufferers feel their pain. Yet studies done on the muscles have not proven that the pain is coming from the muscles. For one thing, researchers have not found evidence of any inflammation in the muscles, but they have found other abnormalities. Biopsies of FMS patients' muscles studied by Bengtsson have shown low levels of ATP, ADP, and phosphocreatine. These are substances our bodies use for energy and they come from the breakdown of food. The distribution of oxygen in our muscles was found to be uneven by Lund, and a low exercising blood flow was also noted by Sharon Clark's group. FMS sufferers will tell you they don't have much of an aerobic capacity while exercising, and this was found to be true when Bennett tested FMS patients' aerobic capacity. An erratic breathing pattern was found by Goldstein in one-fourth of FMS patients studied and would account for the shortness of breath some FMS sufferers experience.

Researchers have found a reduced grip strength in FMS patients, which is a reflection of the weakness many FMS patients report. Researchers do not feel the weakness is coming from the muscles themselves, but could be coming from a dysfunction in the central nervous system. Kristin Thorson has stated in the *Fibromyalgia Network* that some researchers believe we have a heightened response to muscle microtrauma which normally occurs after unaccustomed exercise and causes pain and tenderness 24 to 48 hours after exercising. Another study by Jacobsen has found low levels of the chemical procollagen-type III aminoterminal peptide in the serum of FMS patients which could suggest a decrease in the rate of muscle tissue repair. Researcher Robert Bennett, M.D., has found phosphodiester peaks in 100% of FMS patients' muscles, which is a phenomenon that usually occurs only in elderly patients.

Researchers are suggesting that the abnormalities of muscles in FMS patients are a result of having FMS and not the cause of FMS.

Amino Acids

▲ **Building blocks of protein**
▲ **Used in important processes in the body**
▲ **Must be present in balanced amounts**
▲ **Researchers found low levels of 7**
▲ **Tryptophan needed for serotonin production**

Amino acids are the building blocks of protein which we get from the breakdown of food and are used in various important processes in our bodies. These compounds must be present in balanced amounts in our bodies, and if they are not, many malfunctions can occur. I. Jon Russell, M.D., found low levels of tryptophan, as well as six other amino acids in the serum of FMS patients. Tryptophan is needed to produce serotonin, which we already know is low in FMS patients. In a study by Harvey Moldofsky, M.D., a sleep researcher, when tryptophan was given to FMS patients to see if it would help improve their symptoms, it helped them sleep better, but made their pain worse. Tryptophan is no longer available over the counter in the United States because of a contaminated batch that is believed to be the cause of many people developing a serious condition called Eosinophilia Myalgia Syndrome. Dr. Russell has presented some studies which show that the conversion of tryptophan to serotonin might be dysregulated and could be the cause of some of our symptoms. For an understanding of Dr. Russell's theory on this, please refer to the April 1994 *Fibromyalgia Network,* published by Kristen Thorsen, pp. 3-5. Mohammed Yunus, M.D., found low levels of five amino acids in his study: histidine, methionine, tryptophan, leucine and isoleucine. Supplementing with these amino acids has not yet been researched.

Magnesium

▲ **Necessary for energy-producing activities in the cells.**
▲ **Helps the smooth muscles of the body relax**
▲ **Increases blood circulation**
▲ **Need a red blood cell magnesium test**
▲ **Supplementation**
▲ **Side effects**

Magnesium is necessary for all energy-producing activities in the cells. It helps the smooth muscles of the body relax and also increases blood circulation. A regular magnesium blood test will usually not show a deficiency in FMS patients' cells, but a red blood cell magnesium test will confirm if their level is low. Red blood cell magnesium levels were tested by Thomas Romano, M.D. He found low levels in some FMS patients and then supplemented these patients with oral magnesium–800 to 1200 mg. a day and/or magnesium intramuscular injections. (The patient's dosage was based on his/her specific deficiency.) Some improvement was noted by patients, although it sometimes took weeks or months to feel a difference. The newer forms of magnesium, magnesium glycinate, magnesium aspartate, and magnesium chloride, seem to be better tolerated and better absorbed. Magnesium in high doses can cause diarrhea, so it is important to discuss supplementing your diet with magnesium with your doctor. Another supplement to try is one that contains a combination of magnesium and malic acid. Some health food stores carry a supplement like this, or you can order it. One of these supplements is called FIBRO-CARE and can be ordered from *To Your Health,* a resource listed in the back of this book. A 1200 mg. dose of malic acid has been suggested for daily use. If you would like more information on nutritional aspects for FMS, please refer to the chapter on diet and nutrition.

Brain Scans

▲ **BEAM, SPECT and PET scans**
▲ **Expensive tests**
▲ **Found marked reduction in blood flow**

Doctors are using sophisticated, expensive brain scans like the SPECT scan to target areas of brain dysfunction in FMS patients. Jay Goldstein, M.D., found a marked reduction in blood flow to the right hemisphere of the brain. Another researcher, James Mountz, M.D., found a decreased blood flow to the caudate nuclei section, which has connections to the brain's limbic system and may be involved in memory/concentration problems and pain regulation. The higher the pain score was, the more the blood flow was reduced. Patients with chronic headaches were tested by Thomas Romano, M.D., who found differences in the blood flow between the right and left hemispheres. It may be that the cause of FMS is indeed in our heads! If you are experiencing severe cognitive deficits, your doctor might order one of these scans for you. There are some medications designed to help improve this problem, and you and your doctor can determine if these would be helpful for you to try.

Immune System

▲ **Low natural killer cell activity**
▲ **Abnormal secretion of interleukin-2**
▲ **Low secretion of interleukin-1**
▲ **High incidence of immune reactive protein in the skin**

The immune system may be compromised in FMS sufferers. Natural killer cells seek out and destroy foreign invaders in our bodies. When FMS patients' natural killer cells were tested by I. Jon Russell, M.D., they were found to be in normal amounts, but their activity was low. Researchers do not know why this is so, but serotonin may influence the activity of these natural killer cells. Wallace has also found an abnormal secretion of interleukin 2, a cytokine (chemical) produced by the immune system which fends off infectious agents. When these cytokines are produced by the immune system, they can produce symptoms of pain and fatigue. Dr. Russell found a decreased production of interleukin-1 at the hypothalamic level of control. This chemical increases the secretion of growth hormone, corticotrophin releasing hormone (adrenals), serotonin, norepinephrine and epinephrine, and the beta-endorphins. Beta-endorphins have pain-relieving properties. A high incidence of immune-reactive proteins have been found in the skin of FMS patients. These are not normally seen in a healthy person's skin. In other words, proteins are leaking through the blood vessel walls and accumulating in surrounding tissues, which often occurs in conditions that have an immunologic component.

Sleep and Stress

▲ **Affect immune system adversely**

Some researchers believe an alteration in sleep can contribute to a problem with the immune system, or a disorder with the immune system could be causing a problem with the sleep cycle. (The sleep cycle irregularities are covered in the section on "Sleep.")

Limbic System

Limbic System Dysregulation

Hypothesis: Jay Goldstein, M.D.

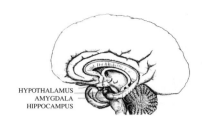

HYPOTHALAMUS
AMYGDALA
HIPPOCAMPUS

Controls

- ▲ Body temp
- ▲ Metabolic rate
- ▲ Memory
- ▲ Fatigue
- ▲ Appetite

- ▲ Immune system
- ▲ Pain
- ▲ Sleep
- ▲ Concept formation
- ▲ Autonomic nervous system

Triggering Event

- ▲ Physical trauma
- ▲ Virus
- ▲ Emotional stress

- ▲ Toxins
- ▲ Infection
- ▲ Childbirth

Treatment

- ▲ Antiviral meds
- ▲ Neurological meds
- ▲ Immune system enhancers

- ▲ Cognitive behavioral therapy
- ▲ Stress management

Dr. Goldstein has been involved in chronic fatigue syndrome and FMS research and believes the two syndromes overlap. He believes the limbic system could possibly be involved in the cause of FMS. The limbic system is a portion of our brain which includes the amygdala, hippocampus and the hypothalamus. It controls body temperature, metabolic rate, memory, learning, fatigue, appetite, autonomic nervous system, sex drive, endocrine system, immune system, pain, sleep, concept formation, blood formation, and others. He believes people are predisposed to developing FMS or chronic fatigue and a triggering event such as a virus, infection, surgery, toxin, childbirth, or severe emotional stress could set off a series of events in the limbic system which could lead to FMS and/or chronic fatigue. If his theory is correct, it may explain the variety of symptoms found in FMS patients because different structures could be affected in different people–producing one symptom such as depression in one person and severe allergies in another, yet both would have pain. On a positive note, he believes these can be treated with antiviral medications, neurological medications and immune system enhancers, depending on each person's symptoms. Since our mental attitudes affect limbic structures, he also believes these conditions can be treated with cognitive behavioral therapy and stress management techniques. His book is listed in the resource section at the back of our book. Dr. Goldstein's protocol is discussed in our section on pioneering treatments and included in the appendix.

RESEARCH

Genetic Studies

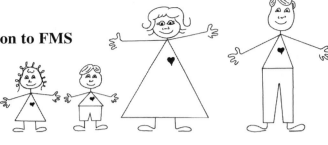

- ▲ **Does FMS run in families?**
- ▲ **Some evidence for a predisposition to FMS**
- ▲ **Studies are being done to determine the possibility**

In one study by Mark Pellegrino, M.D., 50% of the children of FMS patients developed FMS. Another study by Waylonis and Heck reported that 12% of their FMS patients studied had symptomatic children and 25% had symptomatic parents. Many FMS patients report having relatives who had undiagnosed aches and pains, or who after receiving a diagnosis themselves, alert other relatives who then find out they have FMS, too. This is an area of research which is being further studied by M.B. Yunus, M.D., and others and will certainly be of help in putting the puzzle together.

Summary
Research = Cure

- ▲ **More physicians interested in research**
- ▲ **NIH appropriated funds for research**
- ▲ **Write letters to Congress**

In the last fifteen years, FMS has become the focus of research and interest for a handful of physicians. The physicians interested in FMS are to be applauded for their dedication and belief in a condition which frustrates both patients and doctors alike. In fact, there are still doctors who do not believe in the diagnosis of FMS. Fortunately, for us, more doctors are becoming aware of the disorder and are diagnosing it. As more research is carried out, and more doctors become interested in FMS, knowledge will grow and treatments will become more advanced. We will all feel better!

$ = CURE

In the fall of 1993, the National Institute of Health appropriated $1.4 million for FMS research. Never before has there been this much money allocated for FMS research. It is very important for all FMS sufferers to let their congressmen/women know how this syndrome has adversely affected their lives. The research money was given because of the letters and calls FMS patients made to their congressmen/women. Your continued support will help ensure further funding for FMS as progress cannot be made without funds for research. Please write!

RESEARCH

REFERENCES

Ahles, T.A., Yunus, M.B. Riley, S.D., Bradley, J.M., and Masi, A.T. Psychological factors associated with primary fibromyalgia syndrome. *Arthritis Rheum,* 27:1101-1106, 1984.

Ahles, T.A., Yunus, M.B., and Masi, A.T. Is chronic pain a variant of depressive disease? The case of primary fibromyalgia syndrome. *Pain,* 29:105-111, 1987.

Bengtsson, A., et al. Reduced high energy phosphate levels in the painful muscles of patients with primary fibromyalgia. *Arthritis Rheum,* 29 (7):817-821, 1986.

Bennett, R., et al. Low levels of somatomedin-c in patients with FMS. *Arthritis Rheum,* 35 (10):1113-1116, 1992.

Bennett, R.M. (ed) The fibrositis/fibromyalgia syndrome. Current issues and perspectives. *Am J Med,* 1986:81 (suppl 3A):1-115.

Bennett, R., et al. Aerobic fitness in patients with fibrositis. *Arthritis Rheum,* 32 (4):454-460, 1989.

Bennett, R.M., Clark, S.R., Burckhardt, C.S., Walcz, K.J. A double blind placebo controlled study of growth hormone therapy in FMS. *Journal of Musculoskeletal Pain,* (3)1:110, 1995.

Bonafede, P., Nilson, D., Clark, S., et al. Exercising muscle blood flow in patients with fibrositis: a xenon clearance study. *Arthritis Rheum,* 31 (suppl): S14, 1987.

Buchwald, D., Sarrity, D. Comparison of patients with chronic fatigue syndrome, fibromyalgia, and multiple chemical sensitivities. *AMA Intern Med,* 154(18):2049-53, 1994.

Burckhardt, Carol, et al. FMS and quality of life: A comparative analysis. *J Rheumatology,* 20:(3) 475-479, 1993.

Campbell, S.M., Clark, S., Tindall, E.A., Forehand, M.E., and Bennett, R.M. Clinical characteristics of fibrositis. A "blinded" controlled study of symptoms and tender points. *Arthritis Rheum,* 26:817, 1983.

Caro, X.J., Kinstad, N.A., Russell, I.J., and Wolfe, F. Increased sensitivity to health related questions in patients with primary fibrositis syndrome. *Arthritis Rheum,* 30:63, 1987 (Abstract).

Caro, X.J., Wolfe, F., Johnston, W.H., and Smith, A.L. A controlled and blinded study of immunoreactant deposition at the dermal-epidermal junction of patients with primary fibromyalgia. *J Rheum,* 13:1086, 1986.

Clark, S., Campbell, S.M., Forehand, M.E., Tindall, E.A., and Bennett, R.M. Clinical characteristics of fibrositis. II. A "blinded," controlled study using standard psychological tests. *Arthritis Rheum,* 28:132-137, 1985.

Clauw, Daniel, et al. Abnormal auditory event: related potentials in FMS. Abstract. ACR Meeting 1994. Minneapolis, Minn.

Clauw, Daniel, Fibromyalgia: More than just a musculoskeletal disease. *Amer Family Physician,* 52(3):843-851, 1995.

Crofford, Leslie J., et al. Analysis of circadian plasma ACTH and cortisol levels in patients with fibromyalgia (FM) and chronic fatigue syndrome (CFIDS). 1487, Scientific abstracts from the American College of Rheumatology Annual Meeting, October 1996.

Dailey, P.A., Bishop, G.D., Russell, I.J., and Fletcher, E.M. Psychological stress and the fibrositis/fibromyalgia syndrome. *J. Rheumatol,* 17:1380, 1990.

Ferraccioli, Neuroendocrinologic findings in FMS. *J. Rheumatology,* 17 (7):869-873, 1990.

Goldstein, J. *CFIDS: The Limbic Hypothesis.* Haworth Medical Press, New York, 1993.

Griep, E.N., Boersma, J.W., de Kloet, E.R. Pituitary release of growth hormone and prolactia in the primary fibromyalgia syndrome, *J Rheum,* 21(11):2125-30, November 1994.

Hellstrand, K., and Hermodsson, S. Role of serotonin in the regulation of human natural killer cell cytotoxicity. *J Immunology,* 139: 869, 1987.

Hudson, J.I., Hudson, M.S., Pliner, L.F., et al. Fibromyalgia and major affective disorder: A controlled phenomenology and family history study. *Am J Psychiatry,* 142:441-446, 1985.

RESEARCH

Jacobsen S., et al. Primary Fibromyalgia: Clinical parameters in relation to serum procollagen type III aminoterminal peptide. *Br J Rheumatology,* 29 (3):174-177, 1990.

Jeschonneck, M., and Sprott, H., et al. Pathological changes in peripheral blood flow in fibromyalgia, 1484, Scientific Abstracts from the ACR annual meeting.

Johansson, G., et al. Cerebral Dysfunction in FMS: evidence from regional blood flow measurements, otoneurological tests and cerebro spinal fluid analysis, *Acta Psychiatr Scand*, 91(2):86-94, 1995.

Jubrias, Bennett & Klug. Increased reasonance in the phosphodiester region of PNMR spectra in the skeletal muscle of FMS patients. *Arthrit Rheum,* 37 (6):801-807, June 1994.

Kirmayer, L.J., Robbins, J.M., and Kapusta, M.A. Somatization and depression in fibromyalgia syndrome. *Am J Psychiatry,* 145:950-954, 1988.

Larson, A.A., Kitto, K.F. Antagonism of nerve growth factor induced hyperalgesia by the substance PNM2 - terminal meatabolete, SP(1-7). *Journal of Musculoskeletal Pain*, 3(1):1995.

Lund, N., et al. Muscle tissue oxygen pressure in FMS. *Scand J Rheumatology,* 15:165-173, 1986.

McCain, G. Diurnal hormone variation in FMS. *J. Rheum,* 16 (suppl 19):154-157, 1989.

Mengshoel, A., et al. Muscle strength and aerobic capacity in FMS. *Clin Exp Rheumatology,* 8:475-479, 1990.

Moldofsky, H., and Warsh, J.J. Plasma tryptophan and muskuloskeletal pain in nonarticular rheumatism ("fibrositis syndrome"). *Pain,* 5:65, 1978.

Mountz, J., et al. Regional cerebral blood flow in caudate nuclei is associated with pain thresholds in patients with FMS. *ACR 57th Annual Scientific Abstracts of Arthritis Rheum,* S221, 1993.

Neeck, G., Riedel, W. Thyroid function in patients with FMS. *J. Rheumatology,* 19 (7):1120-2, 1992.

Neeck, G., Riedel, W. Neuromediator and hormonal pertubations in fibromyalgia syndrome: results of chronic stress? *Baillieres Clin Rheumatol.,* 8(4):763-75, November 8, 1994.

Payne, T.C., Leavitt, F., Garron, D.C., et al. Fibrositis and psychological disturbance. *Arthritis Rheum,* 25:213-217, 1982.

Pellegrino, M., et al. Familial occurrence of primary fibromyalgia. *Arch Phys Med Rehab,* 70:61-63, 1989.

Romano T.J. Brain SPECT findings in FMS patients with headache. *ACR 57th Annual Scientific Abstracts of Arthritis Rheum,* S250, 1993.

Romano, T.J. Magnesium deficiency in fibromyalgia syndrome. *Journal of Nutritional Medicine,* 4:165-167, 1994.

Russell, I., Vaeroy, H., et al. Cerebrospinal fluid (CSF) biogenic amine metabolites in FMS and rheumatoid arthritis. *Arthritis Rheum,* 35 (5):550-556, 1992.

Russell, I.J., Biochemical abnormalities in fibromyalgia syndrome, *J. Musculoskeletal Pain,* 2(3):101-103, 1994.

Russell I.J. Serum amino acids in fibromyalgia syndrome. *J Rheumatology,* 16 (suppl 19):158-163, 1989.

Russell, I.J., Fletcher, E.M., Tsui, J., and Michalek, J.E. Comparisons of RA and fibrositis/fibromyalgia syndrome using functional and psychological outcome measures. 1989 (Un Pub).

Russell, I., et al. Abnormal natural killer cell activity in fibrositis syndrome is responsive In-Vitro to IL-2. *Arthritis Rheum,* 31 (4 suppl.): S24, 1988.

Russell, I.J., et al. Cerebrospinal fluid substance p is elevated in FMS, ACR 57th annual scientific abstracts. *Arthritis Rheum,* S223, 1993.

Russell, I.J., et al. Cerebrospinal fluid biogenic amino metabolites in fibromyalgia/fibrositis syndrome and RA. *Arthritis and Rheum,* 35 (5):550-556.

Russell, I. Jon, et al. Treatment of fibromyalgia syndrome with super malic: A randomized, double-blinded placebo controlled, crossover pilot study. *J. Rheum*, 22(5):953-8, May 1995.

Russell, I. Jon. *Rheum Dis. Clinics NA*, 15 (1):163, 1989.

Saskin, P., Moldofsky, H., Lue, F.A. Sleep and posttraumatic rheumatic pain modulation disorder (Fibrositis Syndrome). (letter). *Clinical and Experimental Rheumatology*, 2:195, 1984.

Simms, R.W., et al. Lack of association between fibromyalgia syndrome and abnormalities in muscle energy metabolism. *Arthr Rheum*, 37(6):794-800, June 1994.

Sletvold, H., Stiles, T., Landre, N.I. Information processing in primary fibromyalgia, major depression and healthy controls. *J Rheum*, 22(1):137-42, January 1995.

Tanum, L., Malt, V.F. Sodium lactate infusion in fibromyalgia patients. *Biological Psychiatry*, 38:559-561, 1995.

Thorson, Kristin, ed. *Fibromyalgia Network*. p. 6, April 1994.

Thorson, Kristin. *Advances in Research*. Pamphlet, p. 10-11, 1994.

Thorson, Kristin, ed. *Fibromyalgia Syndrome: Advances in Research*. Pamphlet, p. 11, April 1994.

Thorson, Kristin. *Fibromyalgia Network*. p. 6, July 1993.

Thorson, Kristin. *Fibromyalgia Network*. July 1992.

Thorson, Kristin. *Fibromyalgia Network*. October 1996.

Thorson, Kristin. Looking Into Autonomic Nervous System Dysfunction. *Fibromyalgia Network*. October 1995.

Vaeroy, H., et al. Elevated CSF levels of substance p and high incidence of raynauds phenomenon in patients with fibromyalgia. *Pain*, 32:21-26, 1988.

Vaeroy, H., Merskey, M. Progress in fibromyalgia and myofascial pain. *Pain Research and Clinical Management*, Vol. 6: Elsevier Press, 1993.

Wallace, D. Cytokines and immune regulation in FMS. *Arthritis Rheum*, 32 (10):1334-5, 1989.

Waylonis, G.W., and Heck, W. Fibromyalgia syndrome. *American Journal of Physical Medicine and Rehab*, 71 (6), Dec. 1992.

Wendler, Jorg, Hummel, T., Kramer, O., Kraetsch, H., Kalden, J., Kobal, G. Decreased olfactory performance in patients with fibromyalgia in the presence of an increased estimation of subjective sensibility. 380, Scientific Abstracts ACR Annual Meeting, October 1996.

Wolfe, F., Cathey, M.A., Kleinheksel, S.M., et al. Psychological status in primary fibrositis and fibrositis associated with rheumatoid arthritis. *J Rheumatol*, 11:500-506, 1984.

Yunus, et al. Interrelationships of biochemical parameters in classification of FMS and healthy normal controls. *JMP*, 3(4):15-24, 1995.

Yunus, Muhammad B., Rawlings, Karolyn K., Khan, Muhammad, Green, Jack R. Fibromyalgia syndrome (FMS): evidence of genetic linkage to HLA 1482. Scientific abstracts ACR Annual Meeting., October 1996.

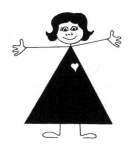

Sleep Disturbance in Fibromyalgia

One of the most prominent features of fibromyalgia is a sleep disturbance. When your head drops to the pillow each night, do you feel as though you spend the next eight hours just skimming on the surface of sleep, hovering in a state of semi-consciousness? Do you get to sleep, but then find that you awaken frequently after the first three to four hours of sleep? It doesn't seem possible that a person could wake up in the morning feeling more tired than when they went to bed the night before, but this is recognized as one of the major symptoms of fibromyalgia.

Five Stages of Sleep

During the night, we normally pass through five stages of sleep in 60- to 90-minute cycles, four to five times per night. These cycles can be traced through the electrical brain waves that occur during sleep, via an EEG (electroencephalogram). The sleep cycles normally progress from very light sleep in stage 1 to progressively deeper sleep in stage 4. Stages 1 - 4 are referred to as non-REM sleep (non-rapid eye movement). During these stages, the electrical brain waves become progressively slower, muscles further relax and the body's metabolism slows. The well rested, restored feeling we get from sleep comes from stages 3 and 4. Stage 5 sleep follows stage 4 and is referred to as REM sleep (rapid eye movement). It is the sleep that occurs when the brain is experiencing increased electrical activity by the neurons in the brain. Your breathing is faster in this stage and your heart rate and blood pressure become irregular. REM sleep is the stage of sleep that is most associated with dreaming. After stage 5, sleep typically progresses through the five stages again, taking 60 to 90 minutes to complete a sleep cycle.

Sleep Disturbance

Many people with fibromyalgia do not progress through these five stages of sleep. They go to sleep easily, but wake up in the early morning (3 to 5 a.m.) unable to go back to sleep or go back into a deep sleep. Others may have difficulty getting to sleep and then have interruptions during the night. Still others may sleep through the night unaware of any sleep difficulties, but may not be experiencing a deep restorative sleep. Similar sleep scenarios are experienced by many people with fibromyalgia.

The sleep disturbance in fibromyalgia that is being described occurs in stage 4 of the sleep cycle. A disturbance in the brain's electrical activity occurs, resulting in arousal, preventing the normal progression through the sleep cycle. The sleep disturbance is referred to by researchers as the alpha-delta sleep anomaly, a condition in which brief periods of awake-like brain waves (alpha waves) interfere with deep level (delta wave) sleep. It can be described as a state of partial wakefulness within sleep itself. When this disruption occurs in stage 4 of the sleep cycle, the body is not restored during sleep. This nonrestorative sleep is believed to be associated with the pain, fatigue and other symptoms of fibromyalgia. While the alpha-delta sleep anomaly is the most common sleep disorder found in fibromyalgia patients, it isn't the only one. I. Jon Russell, M.D., studied 44 fibromyalgia patients and discovered the following sleep disorders: alpha-delta sleep anomaly (43%), sleep apnea (25%), sleep myoclonus (16%) (involuntary arm and leg jerking during the night) and teeth grinding (14%). Another sleep disorder that Harvey Moldofsky, M.D. and colleagues have identified in some FMS patients is K-alpha sleep. This sleep pattern is noted on an EEG and is characterized by brief alpha arousal intrusions, occuring every 20 to 40 seconds. Patients with a K-alpha sleep disturbance have a normal duration of all sleep stages and symptomatically have light unfreshing sleep and daytime fatigue.

Another important component of the sleep disturbance in fibromyalgia involves serotonin, which is the major neurotransmitter essential for the induction of deep level, slow wave sleep. (A neurotransmitter is a chemical that helps nerves transmit their messages.) People with fibromyalgia have been found to have low levels of serotonin in their blood and spinal fluid. At this time, doctors are prescribing medications that increase the availability of serotonin in the body, with the ultimate goal being an improvement in the patient's quality of sleep (more time in delta sleep) and reduced pain sensitivity. More research must be done on the relationship between these medications and the alpha-delta sleep anomaly. While these medications do influence the availability of serotonin, the exact mechanism by which they operate is not understood. There are still many questions to be answered!

Options That May Improve Sleep Quality

If you're waking frequently during the night, discuss with your doctor the option of taking a medication to help improve your sleep quality. (These medications are discussed in detail in the medication section.) If your nighttime awakenings do not decrease after trying a medication for two to three weeks, discuss this observation with your doctor. An increase in dosage, the addition of another medication or a change to a completely new medication may be prescribed.

In addition to medication, listening to a relaxation tape before going to bed can be very helpful for many individuals. Oftentimes patients report that they are able to get to sleep more quickly after listening to a relaxation tape. Some of these individuals also replay the tape during the night, often using headphones, if they're having difficulty getting back to sleep. (There is further discussion of relaxation tapes in the "Stress Management/Relaxation" section in this handbook.) Stress reduction, aerobic exercise and other tips on improving sleep quality (listed at the end of this section) may further help to improve your sleep. We encourage you to try these tips and see what works for you!

Example of Bedtime Routine

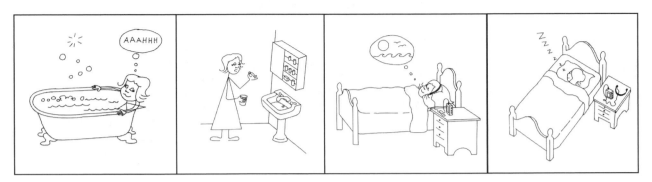

Sleep Log

A sleep log can provide a sample of what your sleep patterns are and how they may vary from night to night. It will be more accurate than your recall and will reflect a general sense of the quality of your sleep. It's helpful for both you and the health professionals working with you to see logs from three to four nights that are sampled over a two to three week period. It may also be beneficial for you to keep additional sleep logs when trying a new medication or implementing a new relaxation technique to document whether or not your sleep improves.

A sample sleep log has been included at the end of this section for your use. An additional sleep log has also been included without the sample, which we encourage you to make copies of and to put in your fibromyalgia journal.

Important Note

Some individuals may experience a sleep disorder called sleep apnea, during which they stop breathing for short periods of time during sleep. If you are concerned that you might be experiencing episodes of sleep apnea and/or would like your sleep patterns further evaluated, we would suggest that you discuss your concerns with your physician. He/she may refer you to the nearest diagnostic sleep center for an evaluation. Patients are often required to spend a night or two at the facility for testing purposes.

Sleep Log

Date	Time to bed	Time of first awakening	Number of subsequent awakenings	Approximate range of time it took to get back to sleep	Time out of bed in A.M.	Medication taken before bed and/or during the night	Comments
Sample 2/15/97	10:30 p.m.	3 A.M.	3	Few minutes to half hour	7 A.M.	Elavil - 9 p.m.	Sleep after 3 A.M. seemed light and disrupted. Sometimes I wasn't sure if I was sleeping or just resting my eyes closed

*Include things that disrupt your sleep and suggestions for improving your sleep.

Sleep Log

Date	Time to bed	Time of first awakening	Number of subsequent awakenings	Approximate range of time it took to get back to sleep	Time out of bed in A.M.	Medication taken before bed and/or during the night	Comments

*Include things that disrupt your sleep and suggestions for improving your sleep.

Sleep Disruption Journal

Check all of the following that are potentially disrupting your sleep. Then write down possible problem-solving strategies for as many of them as you can. You may want to refer to *No More Sleepless Nights* by P. Hauri and S. Linde for some suggestions.

Sleep Disruptions

△ pain

△ need to urinate

△ pets

△ crying babies/children

△ snoring spouse

△ uncomfortable pillow or mattress

△ PMS symptoms

△ menopausal symptoms

△ arguing with family member(s) before bed

△ irregular bedtime schedule

△ stimulant medications

△ eat large meal late

△ inside and/or outside noises

△ too much light

△ uncomfortable temperature in bedroom

△ worries

△ napping too late

△ caffeine

△ alcohol

△ nicotine

△ exercise too late

Problem-solving strategies

TIPS for Improving Sleep Quality

▲ Consult with your doctor about the necessity of taking a medication to improve your sleep quality.

▲ If you are experiencing morning grogginess while taking a medication to improve your sleep quality, take the medication as early as 6 p.m.

▲ Take time to wind down before bed.

▲ Follow a bedtime ritual (e.g., warm bath, listening to relaxing music, reading and other relaxing activities).

▲ Eliminate caffeine after 12 Noon.

▲ Reduce or eliminate fluid intake after 6 p.m. if you have a need to urinate during the night. Medications such as diuretics and blood pressure medications that get rid of excess fluid should be taken earlier in the day, whenever possible. (You will need to consult with your physician first.)

▲ Use relaxation tapes and/or exercises before bedtime.

▲ Develop a program of aerobic exercise, but avoid exercising in the evening.

▲ Actively deal with problems that interfere with sleep (e.g., pain and discomfort, crying baby, uncomfortable mattress or pillow, snoring spouse, concern about safety issues, etc.).

▲ Seek treatment for depression, anxiety and/or stress if you are experiencing these.

▲ Avoid taking a nap late in the day. (It may be more difficult for you to go to sleep at your normal bedtime. Or you may sleep for a few hours, find yourself awake and then be unable to get back to sleep.)

▲ Don't work in your bedroom.

▲ Drinking a glass of milk before bed may be helpful.

Caffeine, Alcohol, Smoking

When you have fibromyalgia, it's important to do all you can do to help ensure good quality sleep. You can begin by reducing caffeine, limiting alcohol, and eliminating smoking.

Caffeine

Caffeine has been shown to cause people to take longer to get to sleep, to cause more awakenings, and to lower their quality of sleep. Individuals vary in their sensitivity to caffeine. For those people who are exceptionally sensitive, it may disturb their sleep after only one cup of coffee or can of caffeinated soft-drink in the afternoon. This sensitivity to caffeine often increases with age. Other symptoms that can be caused by too much caffeine include irritability, nervousness, heart palpitations, dizziness, diarrhea, stomach discomfort and frequent urination.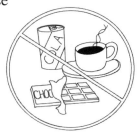

The following tables will help you determine how much caffeine you may be consuming on a daily basis. If you are sensitive to caffeine, try to eliminate it from your diet whenever possible.

Caffeine Content of Beverages and Foods

Item	Milligrams Caffeine	
	Average	Range
Coffee (5-oz. cup)		
Brewed, drip method	115	60-180
Brewed, percolator	80	40-170
Instant	65	30-120
Decaffeinated, brewed	3	2-5
Decaffeinated, instant	2	1-5
Tea (5-oz. cup)		
Brewed, major U.S. brands	40	20-90
Brewed, imported brands	60	25-110
Instant	30	25-50
Iced (12-oz. Glass)	70	67-76
Cocoa beverage (5-oz. cup)	4	2-20
Chocolate milk beverage (8 oz.)	5	2-7
Milk chocolate (1 oz.)	6	1-15
Dark chocolate, semi-sweet (1 oz.)	10	5-35
Baker's chocolate (1 oz.)	16	26
Chocolate-flavored syrup (1 oz.)	4	4

Source: FDA, Food Additive Chemistry Evaluation Branch, based on evaluations of existing literature on caffeine levels.

Caffeine Content of Soft Drinks

Brand	Milligrams Caffeine (12-oz. serving)
Sugar-Free Mr. PIBB	58.8
Mountain Dew	54.0
Mello Yello	52.8
TAB	46.8
Coca-Cola	45.6
Diet Coke	45.6
Shasta Cola	44.4
Shasta Cherry Cola	44.4
Shasta Diet Cola	44.4
Mr. PIBB	40.8
Dr. Pepper	39.6
Sugar-Free Dr. Pepper	39.6
Big Red	38.4
Sugar-Free Big Red	38.4
Pepsi-Cola	38.4
Aspen	36.0
Diet Pepsi	36.0
Pepsi Light	36.0
RC Cola	36.0
Kick	31.2
Canada Dry Jamaica Cola	30.0
Canada Dry Diet Cola	1.2

Source: Institute of Food Technologies (IFT), April 1983, based on data from National Soft Drink Association, Washington, DC. IFT also reports that there are at least 58 flavors and varieties of soft drinks produced by 12 leading bottlers that have no caffeine.

Caffeine Content of Drugs

	Caffeine, milligrams per tablet or capsule
Prescription Drugs	
Cafergot (migraine headaches)	100
Norgesic Forte (muscle relaxant)	60
Norgesic (muscle relaxant)	30
Fiorinal (tension headache)	40
Fioricet (headache pain relief)	40
Darvon compound (pain relief)	32
Soma Compound (pain relief, muscle relaxant)	32
Synalgos-DC (pain relief)	30
Synalgos-DC-A (pain relief)	30
Nonprescription Drugs	
Weight-Control Aids	
Dex-A-Diet II	200
Dexatrim, Dexatrim Extra Strength	200
Dietac capsules	200
Maximum Strength Appedrine	100
Prolamine1	40
Alertness Tablets	
Nodoz	100
Vivarin	200
Analgesic/Pain Relief	
Anacin, Maximum Strength Anacin	32
Excedrin	65
Midol	132
Vanquish	33
Diuretics	
Aqua-Ban	100
Maximum Strength Aqua-Ban Plus	200
Permathene H2 Off	200
Cold/Allergy Remedies	
Coryban-D capsules	30
Triaminicin tablets	30
Dristan Decongestant tablets and	
Dristan A-F Decongestant tablets	16
Duradyne-Forte	30

Source: FDA's National Center for Drugs and Biologics.

Smoking

Nicotine can keep you awake because it's a stimulant. Cigarettes cause a smoker's blood pressure and heart rate to increase and brain-wave activity to be stimulated. Not only do smokers often have greater difficulty falling asleep, but they also tend to wake up more often during the night.

Smoking can be a difficult habit to quit, even if you know that your sleep would likely improve. The rate of success is often better with professional help. You may want to consult with your physician or a psychologist, or try a stop-smoking program recommended by a health care professional.

Alcohol

While many people find that alcohol at bedtime helps them to relax and fall asleep more easily, their sleep is often more disrupted and fragmented. By morning, they've often had less sleep than they would have had without any alcohol. A glass of wine or a cocktail before dinner will likely have less impact on one's quality of sleep, but as with caffeine, people do vary in their sensitivity to alcohol.

Remember to use caution when consuming alcohol and taking medication. This combination may lead to serious side effects, especially with some of the medications used to treat fibromyalgia. For advice on the effect of specific medications and alcohol, it's best to consult your physician.

REFERENCES

Drewes, A. M., et al. Sleep intensity in FMS: focus on the microstructure of the sleep process, *Br J Rheum* 34(7):629-35, 1995.

Drewes, A. M., et al. A comparative study of sleep architecture in subjects with rheumatoid arthritis versus subjects with FMS. *J Muskuloskeletal Pain* 3(1):69, 1995.

Hauri, P., and Linde, S. *No More Sleepless Nights*. New York: John Wiley and Sons. 1990.

Leventhal, et al. Controlled study of sleep parameters in patients with FMS. *J Clin Rheumatol,* 1(2):110-113, April 1995.

MacFarlane, J.G., Shahal, B., Mously, C. and Moldofsky, H. Periodic K-alpha sleep EEG activity and periodic limb movements during sleep: comparisons of clinical features of sleep parameters. *Sleep,* 19: 200-204, 1996.

Moore, K. Sleep disturbances and fatigue in women with FMS and CFIDS. *JOGNN* 24(3):229-233, March/April 1995.

Thorson, K. *Fibromyalgia Network.* 1989, October.

Thorson, K. *Fibromyalgia Network.* 1990, January.

Thorson, K. *Fibromyalgia Network.* 1997, January.

Yunas, M.B., and Alday, J.C. Restless legs syndrome and leg cramps in fibromyalgia syndrome: a controlled study. *British Medical Journal,* 312: 1339, 1996.

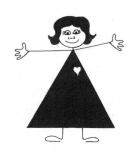

Medications

Why Anti-Depressants? How Do They Work?

These medications have been used for years to modulate pain, sleep and fatigue: symptoms FMS patients can all relate to! Although these medications were not specifically developed for FMS, doctors have found that they seem to help some patients control their FMS symptoms. They may work by increasing the levels of the neurotransmitters norepinephrine, epinephrine and serotonin in the brain. They help us sleep, reduce pain, and elevate mood. At higher doses, they are used for treating depression.

For those of you who have tried many medications that have not worked, it is up to you to seek out a doctor who can help you sort out the problem, or use other techniques such as acupuncture, relaxation, exercise, biofeedback, or hypnosis to control your pain. Hopefully, researchers will find a medication specifically for FMS, and we will all feel better! Until that time, we have to experiment and see what works and what doesn't. It is also important to know that everyone reacts to these medications differently, and what works for you might not work for another person.

You May Need to Try Several

Since each person reacts differently to these medications, you may need to experiment with a few different drugs before you find the one that works for you. Occasionally, these medications can cause in some people the behaviors or feelings they are designed to reduce, for example: depression, nightmares, muscular pain, or insomnia. If these or unusual symptoms occur, notify your physician's office immediately.

Fear of Taking Anti-Depressants

Many fibromyalgia patients are concerned about taking a medication labeled "anti-depressant"–particularly those patients who have been told their symptoms are all in their heads. The chemicals in our bodies that control pain and sleep also control mood, which is why the tricyclic anti-depressants work for some people. If you were depressed, these medications in the low dosages given for FMS patients would not affect your depression at all. They can improve some patients' overall feelings of well-being and reduce pain somewhat, and for those reasons they are worth trying! You could use the example of a diabetic who needs to take insulin every day–we might need the serotonin-boosting effects of these medications just to keep our heads above water! If you become depressed, it is important to have your depression treated. Living with a chronic illness such as FMS increases the likelihood of becoming depressed, so it is important to speak to your physician about treating your symptoms of depression if you do become depressed. Your physician might increase the dosage of your current medication, prescribe another medication, and/or suggest counseling.

Safety

Many FMS patients are concerned about the safety of these medications. When taken under a doctor's supervision, they are safe in the majority of cases. Be sure to report any changes or adverse reactions you are having to your doctor immediately. It is not always necessary to make an appointment with your doctor to discuss side effects or concerns you are having about your medication. A phone call is often all that is necessary. One of the doctor's nurses may also be able to answer your questions. If not, you may ask the nurse to discuss your situation with the doctor and call you back.

It is not advisable to drink alcohol as it magnifies a number of the medication's unpleasant side effects.

These medications can interact with other medications (even some over-the-counter medications), so remember to tell your doctor about all medications you currently use, including cough and cold remedies.

Use Your Pharmacist

Ask your pharmacist questions you have about your medication. He or she is a wealth of knowledge and, if not busy, is often delighted and willing to answer questions you might need answers to. Request the paper insert from the medication box from your pharmacist. It is free and will list side effects, adverse reactions, and drug interactions among other things.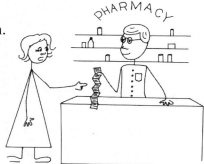

Important Note

You may want to show this section on medications to your physician; this information might help him/her decide what medication would be best for you.

As research continues for FMS, we will find new medications being used in novel ways. Some of these are covered in our section "Pioneering Treatments."

Questions to ask your physician about your medications

1. What dosage? _____

2. When? Morning or Night? _____

3. Possible side effects? _____

4. How long should I try it? _____

5. Do I take it with food? _____

6. Does it interact with any other medications I take? _____

7. Does it interact with any vitamins? _____

8. Can I call the office with questions or do I need to make an appointment? _____

9. What time can I call and whom do I speak with? _____

Comments _____

_____

_____

_____

_____

_____

_____

_____

_____

_____

_____

_____

_____

Medications Most Commonly Used for FMS

Name	Common Dose	Typical Time Taken
Tricyclic Anti-Depressants		
Elavil-amitriptyline	2.5 - 50 mg	in evening
Flexeril-cyclobenzaprine	10 - 30 mg	in evening
Sinequan-doxepin	.25 - 75 mg	in evening
Pamelor-nortriptyline	10 - 50 mg	in evening

May be Prescribed in Small Doses During the Day

Benzodiazepines

(Have Anti-Depressant and Anti-Anxiety Properties)

Name	Common Dose	Typical Time Taken
Xanax-alprazolam add ibuprofen 2400 mg	.25 mg - 1.5 mg - a small dose in morning may be prescribed	in evening
Klonopin-clonazepam	.50 mg - 1.0 mg	in evening

Serotonin-Boosting Medications

Name	Common Dose	Typical Time Taken
Prozac-fluoxetine	1 mg - 20 mg	morning
Zoloft-sertraline	50 mg - 200 mg	morning
Paxil-paroxetine/hydrochloride	5 mg - 20 mg	morning
Serzone-nefazodone	25 mg - 100 mg	morning
Luvox-fluvoxamine	25 mg - 50 mg	evening

Serotonin-Boosting & Tricyclic

Name	Common Dose	Typical Time Taken
Effexor-venlofaxine hydrochloride	37.5 mg	1-2x/day

Sleeping Medications

Name	Common Dose	Typical Time Taken
Ambien-zolpidem tartrate	5-10 mg	in evening

Combination Therapies

Prozac & Sinequan		Elavil & Flexeril
Prozac & Elavil		Paxil & Sinequan
Sinequan & Klonopin		Zoloft & Elavil

These are just suggestions for combinations–

Muscle Relaxants

Name	Common Dose	Typical Time Taken
Norflex-orphenadrine citrate	50 mg - 100 mg	morning & evening or just in evening

Specific dosages need to be worked out with your physician

Medication Dosages

Tricyclic Anti-Depressants

Elavil (amitriptyline) - dose is typically 2.5 to 50 milligrams per night. It is known for its pain-relieving effects and helps you sleep. To avoid morning hangover, take this earlier in the evening or take half your dose in the early evening and the other half at bedtime. You can buy a pill-cutter at your local drugstore. It is easier than trying to break the pills in half or cutting them with a knife. If you feel headed for a flare, you can try taking half your usual dosage in the daytime. Be careful of driving a car if it sedates you too much. This medication has been around for decades and is at this point the medication of choice for many doctors. It may not be effective enough for people who have a high pain level or who have had untreated fibromyalgia for five years or more.

Flexeril (cyclobenzaprine) - dose is typically 10 to 30 milligrams per night. This is a tricyclic drug similar to Elavil, which also has muscle relaxant qualities. If your muscles are in knots, it might prove beneficial to you. It has the same side effects as Elavil. It may be taken in combination with Elavil to provide extra muscle relaxant relief.

Sinequan (doxepin) - dose is typically .25 to 75 milligrams. This is a tricyclic similar to Elavil and functions in the body as an antihistamine. For patients with allergies, it can be helpful. Many fibromyalgia patients have allergies, so it might be worth a try. It comes in a liquid form, as well as in a tablet, which enables you to take smaller doses.

Pamelor (nortriptyline) - dose is typically 10 to 50 milligrams per night. It is another tricyclic that has helped some fibromyalgia patients. It has the same side effects as Elavil, although it may be less sedating.

Other anti-depressants you could try include imipramine, trimipramine, wellbutrin and trazodone. These can be effective for some people. Imipramine and trimipramine are tricyclic anti-depressants. Trazodone is a serotonin specific drug and has fewer side effects than the tricyclics. A low dose would be appropriate to try.

Benzodiazepines (have anti-depressant and anti-anxiety properties)

It is important to note that discontinuing these medications abruptly can produce severe withdrawal symptoms such as tremors and heart palpitations. Be sure to discuss this with your physician before you discontinue these meds.

Xanax (alprazolam) - dose is typically .25 to 1.5 milligrams at night. I. Jon Russell, M.D., has published a study that proves Xanax's effectiveness for fibromyalgia. It has been found to be more effective if taken with ibuprofen (2400 mg./day). For best results you may also need a small dose in the morning.

Klonopin (clonazepam) - dose is typically .5 to 1 milligram at night. It is effective particularly if you have arm or leg jerking spasms as you attempt to fall asleep, which is called sleep myoclonus. If you have sleep myoclonus and you take a tricyclic, it might make you feel worse. It is also good for people with TMJ and those who grind their teeth.

Anti-Anxiety

Buspar (buspirone hydrochloride) - This anti-anxiety medication has not been tested for its effectiveness with FMS patients. You could try it and see if it helps you.

Serotonin-Boosting Medications

Many new drugs are being developed in this class by pharmaceutical companies. By the time this book goes to print, there will be new ones we didn't know about. These new medications may have different effects than the meds already on the market and could possibly work for you. It is important to have a physician who is knowledgeable about developments in this field and who can help you make appropriate choices.

Prozac (fluoxetine) - dose is typically 1 to 20 milligrams in the morning. This is a specific serotonin-boosting drug. If it gives you insomnia, you might have to take it in combination with one of the more sedating tricyclics such as Elavil or Sinequan. It also comes in a liquid form enabling you to take it in very small amounts.

Zoloft (sertraline) - dose is typically 50 to 200 milligrams in the morning. It has been anecdotally proven beneficial for some patients. You may need a sedating medication at night to sleep, as it can cause insomnia or nervousness.

Paxil (paroxetine hydrochloride) - dose is typically 5 to 20 milligrams in the morning. This is another drug similar to Prozac with similar effects. You may also need a sedating medication at night. Paxil is the most potent of these types of medications, and just might have pain-relieving properties for you, as some patients anecdotally report.

Serzone (nefazodone) - dose is typically 25 mg. to 100 mg. daily. This is a newer medication that claims to have fewer side effects than Prozac.

Luvox (fluvoxamine) - dose is typically 25 mg. to 50 mg. at bedtime. This new drug has been approved for obsessive compulsive disorder in the U.S., but has been used to treat depression in Europe.

Other Categories

Effexor (venlofaxine hydrochloride) - dose is typically 37.5 mg. 1 to 2 times per day. The dosage can be adjusted up or down depending on the effects. This is a brand new drug which is not related to the tricyclics or the Prozac-like drugs. It not only boosts serotonin, but has tricyclic properties as well.

Sleeping Medications - These are not used on a regular basis for the treatment of FMS, but may be used occasionally during flares or when you are having severe problems sleeping. You will have to discuss types and dosages with your doctor, since these medications are habit forming. There is, however, a new one called **Ambien**, which Searle drug company claims is less habit forming than other sleeping medications. It is well-tolerated, with few side effects and no known drug interactions. It is available in 5 and 10 mg. tablets. It is not recommended to take it more than two or three times a week. In a clinical trial Searle undertook, they state that FMS patients with sleeplessness reported significant sleep improvement and significantly fewer awakenings.

Combination Therapies - Some physicians are getting good results using various combinations of drugs, such as **Prozac & Sinequan, Prozac & Elavil, Sinequan & Klonopin, Elavil & Flexeril, Paxil & Sinequan, and Zoloft & Elavil.** These are only a few possible combinations. Your doctor will be the best judge of those combinations which will work for you.

Muscle Relaxants - Some physicians prescribe muscle relaxants for FMS patients to take on a limited basis. One to try, particularly if you do not respond to Elavil or Flexeril, is **Norflex (orphenadreine citrate). The typical dose is 50 to 100 mg. 2 times a day.** This medication is a central acting analgesic muscle relaxant that was found by M. Abeles to decrease pain in some FMS patients. It is often taken at night, but some people can tolerate it in the morning as well. There are other muscle relaxants to try if these do not work. Discuss these with your doctor.

NSAIDS - These are the anti-inflammatories such as Motrin, Voltaren, Clinoril, Naproxen, etc. In a study by M. Yunus, these medications when used alone have not been proven effective in reducing pain of FMS, but in a study by I. Jon Russell, M.D., Xanax's effectiveness was increased with the addition of ibuprofen (2400 mg. a day). In another study, Don Goldenberg, M.D. found that Elavil's effectiveness was also improved with the addition of ibuprofen. If you are currently taking large amounts of these, without one of the anti-depressants, you could try stopping them to see if you feel any different. If you have arthritis, osteoarthritis, or tendinitis, they of course would be useful in alleviating that pain.

Toradol - An oral anti-inflammatory drug released in 1992. It has been used in injectable form following surgery and is believed to be as effective as Demerol (100 mg.) without side effects. It may be helpful during flares.

Ultram (tramodol) - dose 50 to 100 mg. every 4 to 6 hours (not to exceed 400 mg. in 24 hours). A pain-relieving medication whose mode of action is not completely known. It does inhibit the reuptake of norepinephrine and serotonin and binds to pain-relieving receptors. Since its use, there have been adverse reports of seizures in susceptible individuals. One of its benefits is that it is non-addictive.

Side Effects

Tricyclic Anti-Depressants

▲ **Morning hangover**
▲ **Constipation**
▲ **Weight gain**
▲ **Drowsiness**

▲ **Heart rate abnormalities**
▲ **Dry mouth and eyes**
▲ **Headache**
▲ **Increased sensitivity to sunlight**

Most of the tricyclic anti-depressants have side effects which are intolerable for some people, such as morning hangover, constipation, weight gain, drowsiness, heart rate abnormalities, dry mouth and eyes, headache and increased sensitivity to sunlight. You can try taking these medications earlier in the evening to avoid early morning hangover. For constipation, eat high-fiber foods (All-Bran works great) and take a daily dose of a natural bulk laxative. Drinking water or sucking on hard candy alleviates dry mouth in some cases. Weight gain is difficult to deal

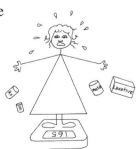

with and many patients find they cannot lose weight no matter what they do. You might also become more sensitive to the sun, so be sure to wear sunscreen.

These side effects generally get better after you have been on the drug for a few weeks. **If not, ask your doctor if you can try a different medication.**

Benzodiazipines (have anti-depressant and anti-anxiety properties)

▲ **Drowsiness**   ▲ **Muscular weakness**
▲ **Impaired coordination**   ▲ **Addictive properties**
▲ **Impaired memory and concentration**   ▲ **Depression**

These medications have anti-depressant and anti-anxiety properties. They can cause drowsiness, impaired coordination, impaired memory, muscular weakness, depression and they have addictive properties.

Xanax (alprazolam) has been shown to be addictive and can cause depression in certain people. I. Jon Russell, M.D., has found that Xanax can be very effective for fibromyalgia if taken in low doses.

Klonopin (clonazepam) is another drug in this class which stays active in the body longer and has the same addictive possibility as Xanax does. It can also cause depression in certain people.

Serotonin-Boosting Medications

▲ **Stomach distress**   ▲ **Mood swings in a small %
                                    of people**

▲ **Anxiety/nervousness**   ▲ **Headache**
▲ **Insomnia**   ▲ **Sexual difficulties**

Prozac (fluoxetine) - This medication can cause insomnia in many patients, therefore it usually needs to be taken in the morning. It might have to be taken in combination with a tricyclic anti-depressant with sedating qualities at night to help you sleep. It can also cause nausea, nervousness, weight loss, headaches and sexual difficulties.

Controversy about Prozac: Following accusations that Prozac caused suicidal behavior in patients, the FDA, The American Psychiatric Association and the National Mental Health Association dispelled these beliefs and pronounced Prozac to be a safe medication.

You must remember that any of these medications can cause abnormal behaviors, but it is a rare occurrence when it happens. Report any bizarre feelings or strange behavior to your doctor immediately.

Zoloft (sertraline) - This drug was manufactured to compete with Prozac. It has similar properties and therefore usually is taken in the morning. It may need to be taken in combination with a tricyclic antidepressant with sedating qualities at night to help you sleep.

Paxil (paroxetine) - Many patients report having less side effects with Paxil as compared to Prozac. It can cause nervousness, sweating, insomnia, nausea and sexual difficulties. Halving the dosage or different timing could help with some of these side effects.

Serzone (nefazodone) - Side effects are generally the same as others, but the drug company claims people seem to suffer less side effects. It may slightly affect memory and cognitive function.

Luvox (fluvoxamine) - Side effects can include headache, weakness, body aches, nausea, palpitations, diarrhea, constipation, drowsiness, insomnia, dry mouth, nervousness, dizziness, sweating, flu-like symptoms, delayed ejaculation, and vomiting.

Other Categories

Effexor (venlofaxine hydrochloride) - The typical side effects when used for its anti-depressive qualities are increased blood pressure, anxiety, nervousness, and insomnia.

Muscle Relaxants - These can make you very groggy, so it is important to take these when you do not need to be alert. If they make you too sleepy, try halving the dose and see if it works better for you.

NSAIDS - These are the non-steroidal anti-inflammatories such as Motrin, Advil, Naproxen, Relafen, etc. These can cause stomach distress, and some patients develop bleeding ulcers from the use of these. There are some newer ones that claim not to produce as much stomach distress. Ask your doctor about them.

Ultram (tramodol) - The side effects may include seizures, dizziness, drowsiness, nausea, constipation, sweating and pruritus. It may also cause sleepiness or be stimulating to some people.

Important Note

Many of the medications may take up to two weeks or longer to work. If there isn't any improvement after one month, ask your doctor if you can increase or decrease the dosage, or try one of the other medications. If your doctor won't allow you to switch, it might be time to switch doctors.

Medication Dosage, Timing and Treatment During Flares

▲ **FMS changes from day to day**
▲ **So can your medications**

▲ **Consult your physician**

Because FMS does have flares and remissions and tends to change from day to day, it is very important to talk to your doctor about increasing your medication during a flare. It is also very important to make sure your increased pain or new pain is actually related to your FMS and not some other medical problem that requires different medical attention. It might help you feel better if you know in advance that it is okay, with your physician's approval, to add an extra dose of a muscle relaxant, increase your regular medication, take more NSAIDS or add a sleeping pill for a few days, depending on your circumstances. Many

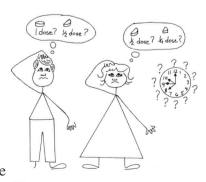

women need to add more medication premenstrually because they tend to have a flare every month at that time. Some people feel worse in the winter when it is colder and the sun is not out as much and could benefit from added medication or light therapy. When physical or emotional stress aggravates your symptoms, this would be another time to add more medication. Talk to your doctor about proper dosages and times of the day when you could benefit from more medication. It will take some time for you and your physician to determine proper dosages and appropriate times to take them, so please be patient.

Options During a Flare

- ▲ **Increase medication**
- ▲ **Add muscle relaxants**
- ▲ **Add a sleeping pill**
- ▲ **Add anti-inflammatory**
- ▲ **Try a topical cream**

Dosages vary from person to person

* Get Physician's Approval Before a Flare Occurs *

Topical Creams

Zostrix cream (capsaicin 0.025%) - This is a topical analgesic you can buy over the counter that is effective for relieving the pain of arthritis in specific areas and has recently been shown to help FMS patients. It is recommended that you use this cream three to four times a day for days or weeks for maximum effectiveness. The actual ingredient in Zostrix or its generic form is capsaicin, which is made from hot peppers. It is absorbed into the skin and actually reduces substance P, which is the neurotransmitter responsible for sensations of pain. It might be useful to try rubbing it in a specific area such as the neck, shoulder or hip to see if it helps alleviate some of your pain. Rubbing it all over your body for fibromyalgia is not recommended. Be careful and follow the warnings on the label. Remember to wash your hands well after applying, because it can be extremely irritating to your eye if you accidentally touch your eye with even a tiny bit of this cream. It can also create a burning sensation (which usually diminishes with time) and can actually burn your skin if you place a heating pad over it. It also may produce a burning sensation if you exercise or sweat, so you might want to wash it off of your skin before exercising or sitting in a hot tub. Other companies have begun to manufacture creams containing capsaicin and they go by many different names. Ask your pharmacist for the brands, as some of these are less expensive than Zostrix. One, called Capsin™, is packaged with a unique applicator so that your hands do not even come in contact with the cream. Another new brand is called Pain-Free™, which is distributed by To Your Health, Inc. (800-801-1406). This company also supplies some other natural vitamin and herbal supplements that have been useful for some FMS patients. They can send you a free brochure. Another type of topical cream is called Aurum® and is composed of methylsalicylate, camphor and menthol. In one study done by Dr. Romano and Dr. Stiller, Aurum helped reduce pain in almost half of the FMS patients. These creams are certainly worth trying! Dr. Phillip Mease of Seattle believes a new cream called Myo Rx, which contains omega 3 and omega 6 fatty acids, is effective in reducing pain levels. Sanford Roth, of Phoenix, Arizona, studied a topical NSAID cream called Hyanalgese-D which was also effective in reducing pain levels.

Important Note

- ▲ **Medications can lose their effectiveness over time**
- ▲ **Try a new one**
- ▲ **Creative prescribing between you and your physician**
- ▲ **Stay in touch for news in drug treatments**
- ▲ **Use a medication diary**

Some patients do not need to take these medications every day, or in the dosages suggested. Sometimes 1/2 or 1/4 the suggested dosage is all that is required every other day or every two days during those times when you are not experiencing a flare. To make it easy to cut your pill in half or quarters, you can purchase an inexpensive pill cutter in the drugstore. Remember, many FMS patients are very sensitive to these medications and sometimes the less, the better. Only you and your doctor can determine what works best for you. It may take some creative prescribing on your doctor's part, but it can be worked out.

If you begin to awaken more frequently at night, discuss with your doctor the option of making a change in your medication. An increase in dosage, the addition of another medication or a change to a completely new medication may be suggested. Postponing this decision for weeks or months, if your sleep continues to be disrupted, may contribute to a flare-up of symptoms.

It has also been reported by Don Goldenberg, M.D., and others, that some of these medications seem to lose their effectiveness after a period of time, particularly Elavil, so it may be necessary to change to another anti-depressant for a period of time to give your body time to adjust. You might then be able to go back to your original medication after a few months and find that it works again.

Summary

- ▲ **Take an active role**
- ▲ **New medications will be discovered**

As more people are diagnosed with FMS and demand effective treatment, new medications to help alleviate symptoms will appear. Researchers are experimenting at this very moment. Since it takes a long time for this information to filter down to you and your doctor, it is very important for you to take an active role in following advances in medication. It would be good if you stayed in touch with a support group, subscribed to an FMS newsletter, attended conferences, and kept in touch with a physician interested in your case.

We have added a medication diary for you to include in your FMS journal. Keeping a written record of your medication, its side effects, dosages and timing will be helpful for you to see how your medication is working for you. It will also enable your physician to make better judgments when prescribing your medications.

▲▲▲

Medication Diary

MEDICATION	DOSAGE	DATE STARTED	TIME TAKEN	COMMENTS*	DATE DISCONTINUED

*Side effects, impact on sleep quality, etc.

TIPS Medication

- Never take your medications without fluids. Take a sip of water first and then the pill.

- One of the possible side effects of the tricyclics could be a dry mouth. A dry mouth for long periods of time can increase the chance of tooth decay, particularly in people with Sjogren's Syndrome, so do not forget to mention this to your doctor or dentist.

- Tricyclics can cause increased sensitivity to sunlight, so take precautions by using a sun block of at least SPF 15.

- Do not put your meds in a medicine cabinet that will be exposed to hot, humid temperatures. It is not wise to leave them in your car or purse where they might be exposed to heat build-up.

- Give up caffeine! It alters and interferes with your sleep pattern. Do not forget that there is caffeine in tea, iced tea, chocolate, and cola drinks. Also, many over-the-counter pain and cold medications contain caffeine.

- Alcohol interferes with your sleep quality and does not mix with these medications.

- Nicotine can affect the effects of these medications.

- If you are just trying a new medication, ask for samples. Many fibromyalgia patients complain that their drawers are filled with unused medications.

- If you cannot tolerate these medications and want to try an alternative, there is a homeopathic remedy called RHUS TOXICODENDRON 6C which has been studied in England and found effective in treating fibromyalgia. There are homeopathic stores available in larger cities, as well as homeopathic doctors. You can call and order it over the phone from Boiron Labs (800-252-0275) and they will send it to you. The cost for a month's supply is about $5.

MEDICATIONS

REFERENCES

Abeles, M. Long term effectiveness of orphenadrine citrate in the treatment of fibromyalgia. ACR 56th Annual Scientific Meeting Poster Presentation. A270, Atlanta, 1992.

Boissevain, Michael D., McCain, Glenn A. Toward an integrated understanding of fibromyalgia syndrome. *Pain,* 45, 227-238, 1991.

Branco, Jaime C., Martini, Alfredo, Palva, Teresa. Treatment of sleep abnormalities and clinical complaints in fibromyalgia with trazodone. 390, Scientific Abstracts, ACR Annual Meeting, October 1996.

Clauw, Daniel, Gaumond, Ethan, et al. Capsaicin skin tests in fibromyalgia. 382, Scientific Abstracts, ACR Annual Meeting, October 1996.

Fisher, Peter. Effect of homeopathic treatment in primary fibrositis. *BMJ,* 229, 365-366, 1989.

Goldenberg, D.L. A review of the role of tricyclic medications in the treatment of fibromyalgia syndrome. *Journ Rheum,* 19, 137-139, 1989.

Goldenberg, D.L., Felson, O.T., and Dinerman, H. A randomized controlled trial of amitriptyline and naproxen in the treatment of patients with fibromyalgia. *Arthritis Rheum,* 29:1371, 1986.

Hales, Ferguson, Yudofsky. *What You Need to Know About Psychiatric Drugs.* New York: Balantine, 1991.

Henriksson, K.G., Bergtsson. Fibromyalgia - a clinical entity. *Canadian Journal of Physiology and Pharmacology,* 69, 672-677, 1991.

Kirsta, Alex. *The Book of Stress Survival.* Great Britain: Simon & Schuster, 1986.

McCarty, Daniel J., et al. Treatment of pain due to FMS with topical capsaicin: a pilot study. *Seminars in Arth and Rheum* Vol. 23 (6) Suppl. 3, pp. 41-47, June 1994.

Moldofsky, M. The effect of zolpidem in patients with FMS - a dose ranging, double blind, placebo controlled, modified crossover study, *J Rheumatology,* 23(3):529-33, 1996.

Romano, Thomas, and Stiller, John W. Usefulness of topical methyl salicylate, camphor and menthol lotion in relieving pain in FMS patients. *Amer Journal of Pain Management,* Vol. 4, pp. 172-174, Oct. 1994.

Roth, Sanford. Topical NSAID therapy in fibromyalgia symptoms in osteoarthritis (OA) with hyanalgese-D, 391, Scientific Abstracts ACR Annual Meeting, October 1996.

Russell, I. Jon. Treatment of primary fibrositis syndrome with ibuprofen and alprazolam. *Arthritis Rheum,* 34 (5), 552-560, 1991.

Russell, I. Jon. Fibromyalgia syndrome: approaches to management. *Bulletin on the Rheumatic Diseases,* 45(3), May 1996.

Searle, Ambien Brochure. July 1994.

Thorson, Kristin. *Getting the Most Out of Your Medicines!* p. 7, 1994.

Thorson, Kristin. Combining science, experience and creativity to treat FMS and CFIDS, *Fibromyalgia Network,* 8, July 1996.

Thorson, Kristin. July. *Fibromyalgia Network,* 1991.

Thorson, Kristin. Prozac-Elavil combination therapy, *Fibromyalgia Network,* 5, January 1996.

Yunus, M.B., Masi. Short term effects of ibuprofen in primary fibromyalgia syndrome: a double blind, placebo controlled study. *Journ Rheum,* 16, (4), 527-32, 1989.

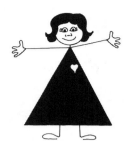

Physical Therapy

Components of a Physical Therapy Program

- ▲ Therapeutic massage
- ▲ Myofascial release
- ▲ Spray and stretch
- ▲ Stretching with heat
- ▲ Heat/Ice/Acupressure

- ▲ Adaptive equipment
- ▲ Footwear ▲ Clothing
- ▲ Aerobic exercise program
- ▲ Stretching program
- ▲ Pacing principles

Many people with fibromyalgia have benefited from these components of physical therapy. A physical therapist can work to help loosen your tight muscles, relieve pain and spasms, increase circulation, promote deep muscle relaxation and improve your range of motion. An important part of the physical therapist's job is to educate you (and a family member or friend, if possible) in those therapies that can be continued at home after your formal physical therapy has been completed. This will include an individualized exercise and stretching program which will help ensure that you are performing the exercises and stretches correctly and safely. (An exercise and stretching program is discussed later in this book.)

It is important to work with a therapist who has recent knowledge and understanding of fibromyalgia. These individuals are best able to evaluate your particular needs and provide the appropriate combination of therapies, while knowing that their services are only one part of a comprehensive approach to your treatment. It is important for your therapist to know where your painful and tight muscles are and to know if his/her touch is too deep or too light. Individuals with fibromyalgia vary a lot in their tolerance for deep massage and degree of stretching. Communicate with your therapist!

In our changing health care environment, we can be sure that there will continue to be changes in the guidelines for physical therapy (including number of visits allowed) and the need for preauthorization. At this time, many insurance companies pay in part or in full for physical therapy if done by a physical therapist with a physician's prescription. Insurance policies do vary, however, so be sure to check your individual policy for specific coverage.

Some individuals with fibromyalgia have additional biomechanical problems that often need to be treated by a physical therapist, either in conjunction with their FMS or separately. A thorough history and assessment by your physician and/or physical therapist will help guide them in choosing the appropriate therapy for you.

Massage

▲ Promotes deep muscle relaxation
▲ Loosens tight muscles   ▲ Increases circulation
▲ Relieves pain and spasms   ▲ Reduces stress

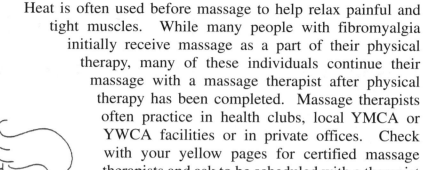

Heat is often used before massage to help relax painful and tight muscles. While many people with fibromyalgia initially receive massage as a part of their physical therapy, many of these individuals continue their massage with a massage therapist after physical therapy has been completed. Massage therapists often practice in health clubs, local YMCA or YWCA facilities or in private offices. Check with your yellow pages for certified massage therapists and ask to be scheduled with a therapist who has worked with clients who have FMS. Full or partial body massages are both usually available, with prices ranging from $35 to $65 for a full hour. Even though massage by a massage therapist is often not covered by insurance, it may be well worth the cost if it helps you to feel better and remain active and productive.

Myofascial Release

▲ Frees up constricted areas
▲ Releases pressure
▲ Relieves pain
▲ Promotes the flow of blood and lymph
▲ Improves range of motion

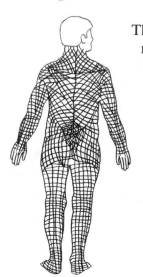

The fascia is a tough connective tissue which surrounds every muscle, bone, nerve, blood vessel and organ of the body. When it surrounds muscle, it's called myofascial tissue. (This drawing illustrates myofascial tissue.) It can be described as a three-dimensional stocking that runs from head to toe. Fascial restrictions often occur in people with fibromyalgia and feel like "knots" or "bands" of tight and painful muscle. The fascial restrictions may be altered by myofascial release. When the therapist has determined where the contracted "bands" or "knots" are in the muscle, he or she will apply gentle pressure in the direction of the restrictions. This gentle hands-on technique can free up constricted areas, release pressure, relieve pain, promote the flow of blood and lymph and improve range of motion.

Spray and Stretch

▲ **Spray skin over tight muscle group**
▲ **Stretch muscle gently**

This technique uses a vapo-coolant spray on a particularly tight muscle group. The spray deadens the pain while the contracted muscle is stretched by the therapist. There are two vapo-coolant sprays available—ethyl chloride and fluori-methane. After receiving instruction on spray and stretch from your therapist, you may request a prescription for fluori-methane from your physician for home use. (Ethyl chloride is not recommended for home use because of its more flammable and explosive nature.) It is helpful to request that a family member or friend also be instructed in this technique by your physical therapist because it is sometimes difficult to do by yourself. Some people object to the spray, especially when it is used on their neck, shoulder and upper back because it's difficult to avoid breathing the vapors. In this case, ice can be used instead to elicit a similar response.

Stretching with Heat

▲ **Apply moist heat**
▲ **Stretch muscle gently**

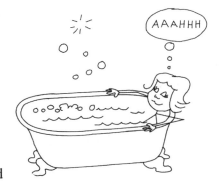

It can also be helpful to use heat before stretching a muscle group. In order to facilitate this stretching, the muscle must be as relaxed as possible. This can be accomplished through the use of moist heat in the form of hot packs, a hot tub or by directing a hot shower on the muscle. Apply the moist heat for 10 to 20 minutes, then gently stretch the muscle until an easy stretch is felt; hold for 10 to 20 seconds or a bit longer and then relax. This technique can gradually help to stretch out the contracted muscle and surrounding myofascial tissue.

Stretching without the use of ice or heat throughout the day can also be helpful, but remember to stretch gently.

Important Note

If you have had recent surgery or have a muscle or joint problem, consult your health care professional before stretching.

Heat/Ice/Acupressure

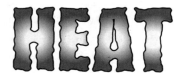

Heat may not only be helpful to use before a massage and before your stretching exercises, but also may be used to aid in relaxation, pain relief and in decreasing muscle stiffness. Microwavable gel packs, heating pads, warm baths/showers, whirlpools, down quilts, long underwear and paraffin baths are examples of various sources of heat. Paraffin baths are designed to be used especially for your hands/fingers. The liquid paraffin has the advantage of applying even heat to all joints of your hands/fingers and can decrease pain and stiffness and increase blood flow. If you choose to use a hot pack, place a light towel between your skin and the hot pack and leave it on the area for approximately 20 minutes.

Important Note

Avoid prolonged exposure to heat sources that could cause burns—check your skin periodically! Do not go to sleep with a heating pad on.

The local application of ice can be used to decrease pain, muscle spasm and swelling. Frozen gel packs, ice packs and packages of frozen vegetables are examples of various ice sources. Place a light towel between your skin and the ice pack and leave it on the area for approximately 10 to 20 minutes.

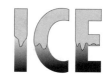

Important Note

Check your skin periodically. If the area being treated turns white or blue, discontinue treatment immediately.

Some people with fibromyalgia have found that by putting gentle pressure on tight palpable bands or knots that they may experience some pain relief. This technique is called acupressure. A thera cane is a device which allows you to independently put gentle pressure on hard to reach places in order to relieve some discomfort. The thera cane is a fiberglass cane which can be ordered from the following address: Thera Cane Co., P.O. Box 9220, Denver CO 80209, (800) 947-1470.

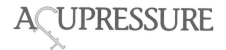

Physical therapy centers and stores or catalogs that sell adaptive equipment also may have the thera cane for purchase. It comes with an easy to follow instructional pamphlet which will help you learn to use it quickly. Remember to use gentle pressure; deep, firm pressure may cause you more discomfort.

Adaptive Equipment

There are many therapy devices being manufactured that can be helpful and are often recommended by physical therapists. These include cervical pillows, lumbar supports, portable massage wands, hot and cold gel packs, portable shiatsu massagers, pen/pencil grips and thera canes. The following catalogs include many of these helpful products and more that can make working, playing and simply living a bit easier. The 800 phone numbers for each catalog are included so that you may call and order a catalog to be sent to your home. Many of these products may also be purchased in drug, department and/or specialty stores. Brookstone is a specialty store found in many local shopping centers that carries a nice assortment of adaptive equipment. Talk with your physical therapist about what items might be best for you.

Adaptability:	**800-243-9232**
Back Saver Products:	**800-251-2225**
Enrichments:	**800-323-5547**
Life Enhancements:	**800-299-0528**
Ortho. Physical Therapy Products:	**800-367-7393**
Saunders Group Inc.:	**800-966-3141**
Solutions:	**800-342-9988**

Footwear

Comfortable shoes with good support and extra cushioning are an important investment for your feet. Both "Easy Spirit" and "Rockport" make excellent walking shoes with extra cushioning to help absorb the shock from walking. Nike, New Balance and other athletic shoe companies also make similar shoes. Socks with extra cushioning may also be a good investment.

If you have a lot of pain when walking on the front part of your foot, or the metatarsus, you may benefit from having a metatarsal orthotic fitted for your shoes. The orthotic will redistribute the weight on your foot when walking and help to decrease your discomfort. If this is a concern for you, discuss this with your physician. (You will need a prescription.)

If you are experiencing a lot of pain in your feet, you will want to consider having your physician or podiatrist further assess them. It's important to find out if a condition other than fibromyalgia is causing your discomfort. Various orthodics or other treatments may be helpful and make walking a less painful ordeal.

Clothing

Dress comfortably whenever you can! Loose knit clothing that is easy to put on and to take off works especially well when you're experiencing a flare-up of fibromyalgia symptoms.

It's best not to wear a heavy shoulder purse on your shoulder for long periods of time. On informal occasions, a fanny pack worn around your waist is an excellent choice.

Aerobic Exercise Program
Stretching Program

Aerobic exercise and stretching are discussed in the chapter on exercise.

Other Therapy Resources and Techniques

Book: *Pain Erasure*

Pain Erasure by Bonnie Prudden gives some helpful tips on how and why seeking massage and myotherapy can help ease painful muscles. This may be a helpful resource for you and assist you in understanding why these techniques can be an important component of your overall treatment program.

Injection and Stretch

Some people with fibromyalgia have areas of tissue that when compressed are tender and produce referred pain and tenderness. These are called trigger points. If these trigger points and other contracted muscle knots are unresponsive to massage, spray and stretch and the other techniques we've mentioned, you might ask your physician to inject these areas with a short-acting local anesthetic. The anesthetic often used is procaine. Temporary pain relief and inactivation of the trigger points injected are possible. Stretching the muscle to its full length after the injection is an integral part of this treatment. A vapo-coolant spray is often used before stretching the muscle. This is followed by the application of hot packs over the injected areas, which helps to reduce post-injection soreness.

Pacing Principles

The importance of pacing is often discussed by physical therapists as they guide individuals with fibromyalgia in developing an exercise and stretching program. Physical therapists also recognize that pacing needs to be incorporated throughout the day in order for fibromyalgia to be successfully managed. Though pacing can be a challenge for many of us, we encourage you to embrace the following pacing principles as you strive for a better balance of work, rest and leisure.

- ▲ Take frequent breaks throughout your day to rest, stretch and relax your muscles.

- ▲ If you need to sit or stand for long periods of time or are working on a lengthy demanding task, take frequent short breaks to change positions and to move around.

- ▲ When you're engaged in activities that include a lot of repetitive movements (e.g., computer work, household cleaning tasks, etc.) you may need to take breaks even more often than usual. A general guideline is to break from a repetitive activity every 20 to 30 minutes.

- ▲ Alternate activities in order to use different muscles and give other muscles a rest.

- ▲ If you're in a car for an hour or more, stop and get out for a short walk and stretch.

- ▲ When you're having a "good" day, resist the temptation to overdo and to work or play with no breaks. Many people with fibromyalgia will pay later with increased fatigue, muscle stiffness, aching and/or pain.

- ▲ Take breaks before you get tired and before you're experiencing increased muscle strain. You may need to set a timer to remind yourself to stop.

TIPS Physical Therapy

- ▲ Physical therapy helps many people with fibromyalgia to feel better. A physical therapist who is knowledgeable about fibromyalgia can help you find the treatment that is best for you.

- ▲ Remember that many times it takes three to four treatments before you begin to feel any benefit. Don't give up too soon!

- ▲ If you experience massage that is too deep for too long or stretching that is too much, you may have a "rebound effect" and feel increased pain and soreness the following day or two. Heat, particularly moist heat, can be very helpful.

- ▲ Remember to ask your physical therapist if you can bring a willing family member or friend to be instructed in massage, stretching and/or spray and stretch. This family member or friend can be invaluable during times of a flare-up of symptoms and for those times that you cannot see a physical therapist, for whatever reason.

- ▲ You do need a doctor's prescription for physical therapy.

- ▲ Most insurance companies do not include massage therapists in their coverage. If you find that massage helps you to remain active and feel better, you may want to have an occasional massage anyway. Your health and well-being are well worth the cost!

REFERENCES

Barnes, J.F. Five years of myofascial release. *Physical Therapy*, 1987, September 16.

Hong, C-Z, Msveh T-C, Simons, D.G. University of California, Irvine, *J Musculoskeletal Pain*, 3(1):60, 1995

Lossing, W. and Boeckman, P. Combining supine cervical distraction with myofascial release and soft tissue stretch for an effective patient treatment. *The American Chiropractor*, 1988.

Prudden, B. *Pain Erasure*. New York: Ballentine Books, 1980.

Sunshine, W. FMS benefits from massage therapy and transcutaneous electrical stimulation, *J Clinical Rheumatology*, 2(1):18-22, 1996.

Travell, J.G. and Simons, D.G. *Myofascial Pain and Dysfunction: The Trigger Point Manual*, 1983.

Weaverman, I. A functional approach to the treatment of fibromyalgia in a physical therapy and stress management setting, *J Musculoskeletal Pain*, 3(1):31, 1995.

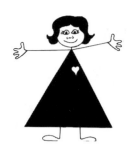

Acupuncture

Acupuncture is a traditional method of treating illness in Asia which has been gaining acceptance in our Western World. It has been used for centuries by Asian physicians for all types of illness and has been noted to be especially helpful in alleviating musculoskeletal pain. A treatment consists of inserting very fine needles in specific points of the body. After the needles are inserted, the acupuncturist might use electrical stimulation, burn herbs or manually stimulate the needles. There should be little or no pain upon insertion of the needles. Once they are in, the patient should not feel them at all and may even lapse into a state of drowsy relaxation. A treatment lasts for 30 minutes to one hour and prices can vary from $40 to over $100. Some of our Western physicians are trained in the technique; many Asian physicians have been using the technique for years. Make sure that the doctor you choose to do acupuncture is licensed and uses disposable needles for your safety.

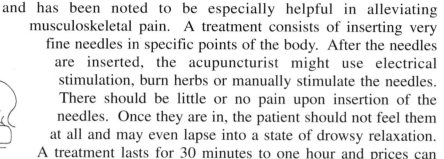

It is not known how acupuncture works. Many believe it helps unblock chi, which is believed to be the life force that drives physical processes and motivates emotions. If chi becomes blocked, imbalances can result in our bodies, causing physical and/or emotional illness. Western physicians believe it works to relieve pain by blocking the pathways that send painful signals throughout our bodies. There have been a few studies done on acupuncture and FMS, and one in particular, using electroacupuncture, showed improvement in over half the patients participating in the study. A few patients felt worse after treatment, however. Acupuncture might be a modality for you to consider as part of your overall treatment plan, particularly if you have not found benefit from medication and other methods of pain relief.

REFERENCES

Blair, James, Mease, Phillip, et al. The use of acupuncture as an intervention in a FMS and CFIDS self-management program. *Journal of Musculoskeletal Pain*, 3(1), 90, 1995.

Deluze, Christophe, Bosia, Lorenzo, Zirbs, Chantraine, Vischer. Electroacupuncture in fibromyalgia: results of a controlled trial. *BMJ* 305:1249-52, Nov. 1992.

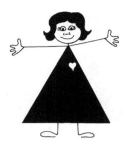

Posture

Good posture and correct body alignment are both important in helping to alleviate undue strain on your muscles, joints, ligaments and tendons. Take a moment to look in a mirror and examine your posture, both standing and sitting. It's important to stand or sit up straight with your shoulders back and your chin tucked in. If you become aware of what your posture and body alignment should be and try to maintain them, you will reduce the stress on your muscles and thereby help relieve the pain and discomfort that occurs from holding muscles in a poor position for extended periods.

Many people with fibromyalgia have muscle aching and pain in their neck and trapezius muscle (a large muscle in the neck, shoulder and upper back). If these same people would assume a forward lean posture (as shown in the illustration) for long periods of time, additional strain would be added to these muscles and their pain and aching would increase. A forward lean posture is easy to assume when working at a desk or computer, especially when you are not at the correct working height. Please refer to the diagram on the right that shows an example of good posture and correct body alignment when sitting at a computer.

Learning to stretch muscles that may have become constricted over time because of poor posture can be important in helping you to maintain good posture and correct body alignment. Bob Anderson's book, Stretching, is an excellent resource for stretching exercises. Self Help Manual for Your Back, by H.D. Saunders, is also an excellent resource for posture, stretching exercises and good back care. A physical therapist can be very helpful in teaching you the correct stretching exercises and can instruct you in good posture and correct body alignment. An occupational therapist is trained to help people restructure their work and home environments to help them maintain good posture and decrease the energy required to do a specific task. Yoga can be a helpful adjunct to improving overall flexibility and strength. It also has the additional benefit of improving your posture! If you have concerns or questions regarding posture, don't hesitate to ask a physical or occupational therapist to evaluate your particular situation.

▲▲▲

REFERENCES

Anderson, B. *Stretching*. Bolinas, California: Shelter Publications, Inc., 1980.
Saunders, H.D. *Self Help Manual for Your Back*. Minneapolis: Educational Opportunities, 1990.

POSTURE

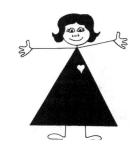

Practical Coping Tips

The following tips are additional ways of coping that we've found to be helpful. Try some and see if they're helpful for you, too. The tips are organized in the following categories: fatigue, family and friends support, memory problems, morning stiffness, and miscellaneous coping tips. You may want to write down other practical coping methods that you've discovered on your own at the end of this section. There are also additional tips at the end of most sections which you will want to read.

Fatigue

Fatigue can be one of the most debilitating and frustrating symptoms for FMS patients. The fatigue you are experiencing is most likely different from any fatigue you have experienced before and may be overwhelming. Some people describe this fatigue as being similar to experiencing constant jet-lag. The levels of fatigue patients experience can range from mild to severe. Some people have enough energy to lead a fairly normal life and others have a great deal of difficulty getting out of bed. Some find they are energetic for a few hours during the day and then a few hours later can barely move because fatigue has overcome them. FMS sufferers often say they feel they have "hit the wall" with their fatigue and can go no further. It definitely can be frustrating. Not knowing when the fatigue will strike is stressful and makes it difficult to plan your daily activities. It is reassuring to know that as your symptoms improve, your fatigue levels should improve as well.

Tips for coping with fatigue

▲ **Plan**
▲ **Pace**
▲ **Prioritize**

Helps to reduce fatigue and pain.

Plan

▲ Speak to your physician about medication to get a good night's rest. Lack of sleep is the major contributor to feeling fatigued.

▲ Use schedules, lists, and calendars. These are also useful for coping with memory problems. You can purchase planners/calendars that will fit in a purse or could be left by a desk. Please do not try to fit too many activities into one day. A "to do" list is great for keeping you reminded of what you need to do each day, but be realistic about the number of items on your list. Cross off each "done" item and see how much you've accomplished!

▲ Plan for a rest period each day. Schedule a longer period of time during the week, an afternoon or even a day if possible, when you can relax and take care of yourself. This is particularly important to have planned into your schedule after you have a busy series of events.

▲ Plan to do an activity that you enjoy each day. We all feel less fatigued when participating in an activity we like doing.

▲ Organize your home so things are within easy reach for you. You shouldn't have to do any unnecessary reaching for items stacked in high cabinets or spend extra time sorting through cluttered closets and drawers. It may take some time to get organized, but it will be worth the effort.

▲ Are you eating well-balanced meals? Lack of proper nutrition robs us of energy.

▲ Exercise. If you do not overdo, it can increase your endurance and boost your energy level. Please refer to the exercise section for help with planning an exercise program.

▲ Plan activities so you have a restful or an uplifting activity after a strenuous one. Alternate these. For example, do not plan to vacuum and scrub floors in the same day. Vacuum, then write those letters or pay the bills. Scrub floors another day.

▲ Avoid errands and/or shopping during busy traffic hours. You will feel less stressed. Shopping during off hours will allow you to spend less time standing in long lines and will save you energy.

Pace

▲ We know how hard pacing is to do and admit that it is a real challenge. It seems we all want to do everything during those times when we feel better, but then feel exhausted from overdoing and send ourselves into a flare! Be realistic about the goals and activities you set for yourself.

▲ Take frequent short rest breaks during the day. Stretch, take deep breaths, or just close your eyes and listen to soothing music.

▲ Use a relaxation tape when you are feeling most fatigued. You may be amazed at how refreshed you will feel afterwards. You might even feel better than if you had taken a nap!

▲ Try to do your heavy or difficult tasks when you know you will have more energy.

▲ Listen to your body. Rest before you get over-tired. Sometimes this is difficult for FMS patients; we are tired all the time and do not even realize when we have really overdone it, until it's too late.

Prioritize

▲ Take care of the important things first. Your stress load might be reduced if you do the tasks you really dislike doing first. This will save you worry time which will alleviate some fatigue caused by worry!

▲ Decide which activities you do not need to do. Which ones can you postpone? Sometimes we do things that might be better left undone.

▲ Ask other people to help you with tasks you find difficult.

▲ Learn to say no. Many of us are over-committed. Weigh what you have to do against what you want to do.

▲ Make yourself and your health a priority.

Family and Friends Support

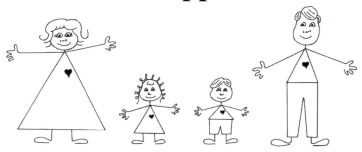

It's often difficult for family members and friends to understand the degree of pain and fatigue that you're experiencing because fibromyalgia is an invisible condition. This scenario may create feelings of isolation and loneliness in you and the belief that "nobody understands." As you struggle with chronic pain and fatigue, you may have a tendency to conserve energy by further isolating yourself. By doing so, you unfortunately may be cutting off the very support that you need in order to live successfully with fibromyalgia.

Take time to inventory your support system. Identify those individuals who are helpful and those who are not. Well-meaning family members and friends do not always possess the ability to give you the kind of support that's really helpful. During this inventory process, also identify those family members and friends who are more supportive and helpful in certain situations. Clarify the strengths and weaknesses of your support network and begin to elicit support from those best able to help you. When you're able, nurture those individuals closest to you; your support network is a valuable asset.

Helpful support suggestions for family members and friends

▲ Even though I look well and don't complain, please understand that much of the time I do not feel well. I am in pain and have overwhelming fatigue.

▲ Please understand when I tell you that I can't go on an outing or engagement. I wish that I could do all the things that I'd like to do.

▲ You are experiencing the loss of a healthy me. Share your feelings about this loss, but please don't be angry with me. I didn't choose to have fibromyalgia. It is not my fault, and I grieve too.

▲ Let's do things together on days when I feel good, or schedule them earlier in the day when I have the most energy. Can we go out to brunch, rather than dinner? Can we celebrate at home?

COPING TIPS

- When we go to the zoo, please understand I need frequent rest breaks. We can have fun and enjoy our times together, but we may have to adapt and do things a bit differently.

- When I'm having a flare-up, please ask me how you can help. Offer me a back rub. Remind me that even though the pain is bad now, it won't last forever.

- Believe me when I say I have pain. So much of the time, I suffer in silence! Tell me you believe me.

- Support me in all I must do to take care of myself—rest, sleep, relaxation, medication, medical care, support and exercise.

- Keep telling me you care about me, affirm my courage and my efforts to get better.

- Recognize that I often feel irritable when I am fatigued and in pain. I don't mean to hurt you.

- Hug me, give me warm touches and loving words of acceptance.

- I appreciate all you do to help support me, even when I forget to tell you so.

- Always remember how important your love and support are to my well-being and my success in meeting the challenges of living with fibromyalgia.

Memory Problems: CRS—can't remember stuff!

Many individuals with fibromyalgia experience cognitive problems. Trying to remember a name, putting the wrong word in a sentence, forgetting what your supervisor just told you to do five minutes ago, misplacing things, an inability to concentrate on reading or studying are common complaints by many FMS patients. Sometimes these problems in cognitive functioning are referred to as "fibro-fog." When fibromyalgia symptoms are flared, often memory and concentration problems will also be more severe. It is not fully understood why this occurs because the brain's processing system is very complex. It is known, however, that poor sleep quality exacerbates cognitive problems. As you get better, your difficulties with memory and concentration should improve. If your cognitive problems are really extreme, discuss these symptoms with your physician. Further evaluation may be necessary.

Tips for coping with memory problems

- Use a desk calendar large enough to write in the activities you need to do each day. Check it every day.

- Make a list of important phone numbers for each phone in your house. Tape it to the wall or inside your cabinet so it doesn't "walk away," preferably right next to the phone.

- Keep a pad of paper next to your favorite chair with a pen to jot down notes to yourself.

- Buy a pocket recording message tape player that you can speak into and leave audio messages to yourself. Don't forget where you keep it!

- Talk to your doctor about your memory problems. He or she can determine if you need medication and/or if depression is contributing to your memory problems.

- Consider seeing an occupational therapist. These health professionals will often suggest excellent memory compensation techniques to use until your memory and concentration improve.

- Exercise your mind. The more you do to use your mind, you may find your memory problems decrease. Do crossword puzzles, try to read interesting articles or books.

▲ Try to avoid taking oral directions when traveling by car. Keep a notepad handy on which to write directions and any other important information you need to remember.

▲ Speak to your family about your memory problems. It will save you some worry!

▲ Don't feel bad when you ask someone to repeat something they just said. Tell them you have CRS (Can't Remember Stuff)!

▲ If your memory is interfering significantly with work, you may need to talk to your supervisor or someone in the Human Resources Department. Explain the specific difficulties that you're having with your memory and ability to concentrate. Oftentimes it's better to get things out in the open. Allow yourself more time for projects at work or make the decision to do some extra work at home.

▲ Avoid stressful situations when you can. They often make memory problems worse.

▲ Leave tasks that require concentrated effort for those times of the day and/or week when you feel better.

▲ Divide tasks into smaller portions. Do a little at a time and they will seem more manageable.

▲ Keep lists! Try to keep your lists in a planner or at a specific spot in your house. For example, on a desk or table in the kitchen or another room you frequently inhabit, such as the family room or den. Some individuals find that Post-It® notes are helpful.

Morning Stiffness

Many individuals with fibromyalgia report experiencing stiffness in the morning when they get out of bed. Muscle stiffness can also reoccur throughout the day, especially after being in one position for an extended period of time.

Tips on coping with morning stiffness

Jenny Fransen, R.N.

▲ Prepare your clothes, lunch, gas up car, etc., the night before.

▲ Choose easy-care clothing and hairstyles. Dress for comfort.

▲ Simplify your morning routine as much as possible.

▲ Always allow extra time to get ready in the morning. Avoid rushing when you are stiff and in pain.

▲ When you get out of bed, take a hot bath or shower to relieve pain and help loosen up muscles and joints, then stretch and do range of motion exercises.

▲ Hot paraffin may help relieve stiffness in your hands and fingers.

▲ Take medication upon awakening to reduce pain. You may even want to set an alarm early to take medication and then go back to sleep.

▲ Whenever possible, adjust your routine to accommodate morning stiffness. You may need to schedule early morning activities later in your day.

▲ Isotoner gloves (turned inside out) have been found to reduce swelling in the hands when worn at night.

▲ Cushioned resting splints worn at night help to reduce swelling, pain, and stiffness in the morning.

▲ Upon awakening, slip on shoes with cushioning, like aerobic or walking shoes. They provide support and cushioning to stiff and painful feet.

▲ Use adaptive equipment with easy grip handles, building them up with adhesive back foam, foam curlers, or pipe insulation. Consider building up tooth brushes, hairbrushes, steering wheel, etc.

▲ Report how long you are stiff in the morning to your physician. This information is important to know in planning your care.

▲ Ask for help from family members. Let them zip back zippers, assist with breakfast, and help with other early morning tasks.

Miscellaneous Coping Tips

▲ Take frequent breaks throughout the day to change positions. If you're sitting for a long time at your job, in a movie theatre, in a plane or car, etc., get up, move around, and gently stretch.

▲ A very hot bath once or twice a day can work wonders to give you temporary pain relief and relax your mind as well.

▲ Take your favorite pillow along on trips. It will save your neck!

▲ Check muscle tension throughout the day–are you tensing your shoulders, holding your breath, or clenching your teeth?

▲ When you have to carry heavy items, use a fold-up luggage cart to make your load lighter.

▲ When you go on a trip, instead of taking one large fully packed suitcase, take two smaller ones. Suitcases with wheels will make your travel plans easier, too.

▲ Invest in one of the electrical massagers that you can lean up against–it can help loosen tight muscles and take your mind off of the pain. It also will not get tired!

▲ Instead of carrying a heavy purse, try wearing a fanny pack to reduce muscle pain in the shoulder area. You could carry your wallet and other necessities in your pockets, too.

▲ Keep a back pillow (lumbar support) in your car to relieve tension when driving. You can buy specially designed ones or place a rolled-up towel between the small of your back and the car seat.

▲ When reading, put your book or magazine on a pillow in front of you to reduce stress in your arms and to assist you in improving your posture.

▲ Shoulder pads can actually cause pain in your shoulders if they are too large. Remove them from your clothing, if necessary.

▲ Make sure bra straps are loose and comfortable. Tight ones can constrict circulation and be painful.

▲ Let your family members help you whenever possible. It is hard to give up activities we have always done, but when you are feeling better, you can gradually do more.

▲ Make sure your work station is at a good height for you. It should not cause stress on your arms or your neck.

▲ Don't apologize for having fibromyalgia. Don't be put on the defensive by "well-meaning" friends or relatives. Learn to say "no" if you cannot or do not want to perform certain tasks. For your real friends no explanation is necessary; for others, no explanation will ever suffice.

Coping Journal

Date	Planning Things to do	Pacing When to do them	Prioritizing In order of necessity

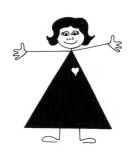

My Battle with Fibromyalgia

Pain and fatigue
have come again
like an enemy
seeking to destroy life.

Like a storm at sea
the waves sweep over me
and threaten to dash me
to the rocks below.

But I have a lifeline.
I know my enemy well
and I know I will win.

I will ride out the storm
knowing that it will subside
and the sun will shine again.

Once more I have won.

Peggy J. Donahue

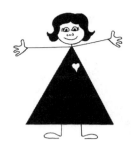

Vicious Cycle of Pain in Fibromyalgia

Some researchers believe a neurotransmitter deficiency is responsible for the sleep disorder associated with FMS. The precise relationship remains a mystery, but continues to be researched. Some believe the muscle pain and fatigue then develop and become worse when you are sedentary or do not exercise. Then if you experience depression, the neurotransmitter serotonin may be further lowered and your sleep becomes more disrupted. Researchers are currently exploring possible causes for the serotonin deficiency. Until a cause is discovered, you may want to try to break the vicious cycle of pain as follows:

Neurotransmitter Deficiency

Depression

Sleep Disorder

Muscle Contraction and Severe Pain

Muscle Pain and Fatigue

Voluntary Immobilization and Muscle Deconditioning

Neurotransmitter deficiency: medication, meditation, nutrition

Sleep disorder: medication, sleeping tips, relaxation, exercise

Muscle pain and fatigue: better sleep quality, medication, relaxation

Voluntary immobilization: physical therapy, exercise

Muscle contraction and severe pain: heat, gentle stretching, massage, medication, acupressure

Depression: medication, counseling, support

If you are depressed, understanding the vicious cycle of pain will help you realize why it's so important to receive counseling and/or medication for your depression to break this vicious cycle. Treating depression is an important part of the overall management of your fibromyalgia.

One of our aims is to help you improve your symptoms and your quality of life. If each part of the treatment plan helps you feel a small percentage better, when you add them all up you can feel over 50% better. We realize we are asking you to make many changes in your life, and we know how overwhelming this can be. We offer these to you as options, and it is up to you to decide whether or not you want to try one change or more than one. They all have the potential to help you, but may affect each individual differently. Exercise might make you feel better, but might make someone else feel worse! It is the same with medication, physical therapy, relaxation, biofeedback, and other treatment alternatives.

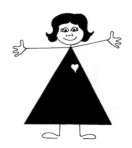

Exercise for Fibromyalgia Patients

Do you remember when you could lift your grocery bags without pain or run up a flight of steps and not get short of breath? Did you attend exercise classes and feel great afterwards? Now do you wonder when you will be able to walk around the block again without feeling as if every muscle in your body is screaming in pain? Yes, your body is not what it used to be! You must accept this reality or you will become frustrated and will not improve! Improving your physical fitness and the way you feel takes

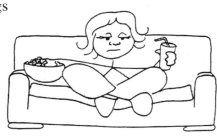

▲ **Guidance**
▲ **Patience**
▲ **Perseverance**

▲ **Determination**
▲ **Time–lots of it**
▲ **Realistic goals**

Some researchers feel FMS patients might have an inherited quality for exercise intolerance. Since we know that the **average** person loses 3% of his/her strength for each day of inactivity, we can only imagine how much strength an FMS patient has lost due to his/her inactivity. Research has shown that FMS patients do indeed have muscle weakness.

Remember

▲ **Do not dwell on the past**
▲ **Start with where you are now—not where you used to be!**
▲ **Don't compare yourself to others**

Try not to dwell on the past–it doesn't serve any purpose except to make you feel bad about the things you can't do anymore. You can learn to substitute activities you can't do with activities you can do. You will need to start with activities you are able to do right now–even if that's only walking to the front door–and increasing your activity level as you are able. It is also very important not to compare yourself to others–you might not be able to do the same amount and types of activities others can do, and this will only frustrate you and make you feel bad about yourself. You don't need that! What you need is to feel good about yourself by honoring your body, treating it with the utmost care and respect, and it will repay you with increased vitality and less pain.

Why Aerobic Exercise?

Several studies have confirmed the effectiveness of aerobic conditioning exercises for fibromyalgia patients. It

▲ **Reduces tender point pain**

▲ **Improves sense of well-being by releasing endorphins into our bloodstream**

▲ **Helps us sleep by making us physically tired**

▲ **Floods muscles with much needed oxygen**

▲ **May activate the immune system**

▲ **May increase serotonin levels**

▲ **Improves self-esteem**

▲ **Reduces depression**

Getting Started

The patients who can participate in some form of aerobic exercise seem to feel better over time, although not everyone benefits. More studies are needed to determine why some feel better when they exercise and others do not.

Some of you might be thinking that you hurt so much that just walking around the block is next to impossible! There are some obstacles you may have to overcome to work up to an exercise program:

▲ **Check with your doctor before you begin to make sure you don't have any joint, muscle or disc problems that could get worse by exercising too vigorously or inappropriately.**

▲ **Get your fibromyalgia under control with medications that might help alleviate some of the associated pain and stiffness.**

▲ **If possible, work with a physical therapist knowledgeable of fibromyalgia problems who can guide you in an exercise program.**

▲ **Approach should be gradually progressive. Over-exercising is to be avoided. It will only make your fibromyalgia symptoms worse.**

The type of doctor who could guide you in an exercise program could be:

▲ **Rheumatologist**
▲ **Internist**
▲ **Physiatrist**

Because fibromyalgia affects each person differently, you may find yourself having to start at the beginning of this exercise program if you have a severe case of fibromyalgia. If your fibromyalgia is not very severe, you could begin at a higher level. If you are already in an exercise program, great! Keep it up!

The key is to start out slowly. Fibromyalgia patients need to start slower and increase their workouts much more slowly than the average person. If you have chronic fatigue syndrome as well, you might find that exercise makes you feel worse. Listen to your body! If you feel really terrible after exercising, cut back. Go slower. Spend more time stretching. If you feel any unusually extreme pain, **STOP** and contact your physician. You may experience some muscle soreness at first. This is normal for fibromyalgia patients. If you keep it up you will gradually increase your ability to exercise with less muscle soreness. In his book The Fibromyalgia Survivor, Mark Pellegrino, M.D., says that you are not hurting yourself by exercising and that the muscle soreness should decrease, so don't be afraid of the soreness.

Aerobic Exercises Beneficial in FMS

- ▲ Walking
- ▲ Bicycling
- ▲ Warm water swimming
- ▲ Nordic Track

- ▲ Treadmill
- ▲ Stationary bicycle
- ▲ Water aerobics
- ▲ Dancing

Pick an exercise you like

It is important to pick an exercise that you enjoy doing. If you hate to swim and your physical therapist encourages swimming, you might not keep it up. Alternating aerobic activities helps keep some people motivated. Bouncing or jarring exercises are not good for people with joint, disc or spinal problems, and may cause additional discomfort and injury. Many people prefer to exercise with a friend or in a class. If you do choose to exercise with others, make sure their level of physical fitness is similar to yours. If they can exercise longer or more vigorously than you, you will have a difficult time keeping up and will only become discouraged.

Before Beginning Your Exercise Program

It is important to remember that you are not training for a sports event. You are training for your health and well-being, so training at 70% of your aerobic capacity may be too difficult. Try to produce a breathless feeling at least twice during your session. We feel it is more important to keep moving than it is to worry about training intensity.

Stretching Is Very Important

Stretch before you begin any workout. Pay close attention to those areas that are problems for you. You may need to spend more time stretching those areas where your muscles are tightest. We have some stretches pictured for you at the end of this section. Some of you might have to spend a few weeks just stretching before you even begin an aerobics program. Because stretching is so important, it is necessary to learn the proper method for stretching. A physical therapist can help; a sports trainer or some videos that incorporate gentle stretching along with low-impact aerobic exercises can also be helpful. A very gentle yoga class could prove beneficial and is a wonderful way to gain flexibility and strength and reduce stress. The book *Stretching*, by Bob Anderson, is available in bookstores for $9.95 and is a good one to add to your collection. It is also helpful to get into the habit of stretching throughout your day. Take frequent stretch breaks when you are working, sitting for long periods, or feel extra tense. Stretch to the point of resistance, hold it until you feel your muscles give, but don't ever force anything–you will only hurt yourself. If you have extreme pain in certain areas when you try to stretch, you might have trigger points which could be helped by trigger point injections. A doctor trained in doing these injections could determine if you might be helped with this form of therapy.

After you are stretched out, you can begin your aerobics program. One important reminder is to keep your arms close to your body when you exercise. This position will help reduce fatigue and pain during exercise, as well as other physical activities such as gardening, sweeping, vacuuming, folding laundry, painting, computer work, etc. Also try to keep any repetitive movement to 20 minutes or less. FMS patients' muscles seem to respond poorly to repetitive movements.

Exercise Diary

It is also wise to keep an exercise diary. We have included a sample page for you to photocopy and use. It will enable you to keep a good record of exactly how much progress you have made and how you feel. If you do not keep a record of your progress, it is often hard to see the gains you have made, particularly if they happen very slowly as so often seems the case for FMS patients.

Exercise Program

- ▲ **Stretch before**
- ▲ **Begin with amount you can do without pain**
- ▲ **Low-impact aerobics**

- ▲ **Increase slowly**
- ▲ **Stretch after**
- ▲ **Target heart rate**
- ▲ **Goal: 20-30 minutes 3 to 4 times a week**

▲ Stretch before every workout.

▲ For beginners: Start with the amount of time you can exercise without fatigue or pain. Try increasing that by two minutes every three workouts. If that produces a lot of pain, back off and increase more slowly–try one minute every week.

▲ One method that works well is to break your exercise time into two times a day. Divide the amount of time you can comfortably exercise by two. Do one half in the morning and the other half in the afternoon or evening. Gradually increase this time until you reach ten or fifteen minutes without pain, and then drop back to one time per day. This method helps to avoid flare-ups.

▲ Stretch after every workout. This is very important.

▲ Some of you ask about target heart rate–if you wish to aim for that goal, the way to figure your target heart rate is to subtract your age from the number 220 and then take 60-70% of the resulting number: 220 - 40 = 180 x 60-70% = 108-126 beats per minute for a 40-year old.

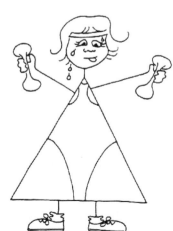

▲ Goal: 20 to 30 minutes three to four times per week. (This time does not include time spent stretching before and after exercising.) If you feel fine after exercising for 20 or 30 minutes, of course you can exercise longer if you like. Just remember, if you overdo it, you will hurt!

▲ You must keep up your exercise routine indefinitely.

It is important for you to remember:

▲ **Improvement time varies from individual to individual.**

▲ **Adjust the intensity of your program according to how your body feels.**

▲ **Modify your workout to include those areas that need to be treated gently if you have specific problem areas.**

▲ **There will be setbacks. FMS has a course of flares and remissions. Don't overdo it when you're feeling better; go easy when you are in a flare.**

▲ **Don't give up!**

▲ **Stretch throughout the day.**

▲▲▲

Exercise

▲ It might take as long as three to six months to see improvement. Remember that fibromyalgia people are not as predictable in their responses, so it is important not to measure yourself against others.

▲ Find a friend to exercise with. It will be more fun and will encourage you to keep it up.

▲ Keep an exercise diary so you do not forget how much you exercised the day before.

▲ Exercise tapes are great to use. Pick a low-intensity one, such as *Low Impact Aerobics* by Jane Fonda, *Starting Out* by Kathy Smith, or *Sweating to the Oldies* by Richard Simmons. There are many others to choose from. It seems that every movie star has produced an exercise video! The Arthritis Foundation offers exercise tapes which would also be great to try. Pace I and II are excellent for senior citizens and wheelchair-bound patients. Some support groups offer tapes–a list is offered at the end of the book. Some tapes also include stretching and gentle yoga exercises which would be useful to try. Some libraries and video stores offer these tapes as rentals so you can try before you buy!

▲ Try to incorporate into your exercise workout the use of all your muscle groups.

▲ Remember that most people who can keep up an exercise routine tend to feel better.

▲ Nautilus weight-lifting machines tend to be too difficult for fibromyalgia patients and may aggravate fibromyalgia symptoms. You might be able to handle them as your strength increases, but don't be upset if you can't. You can add strength training after you are well-established in an exercise routine. Start out with very low weights (1 lb. or less) or try using elastic bands which give a good workout.

▲ Warm water swimming is an excellent aerobics program for fibromyalgia because it is gentle on the joints and the warm water relaxes the muscles. Water temperature must be at least 86°F. Many communities and hospitals have therapeutic pools and classes. You might need a prescription from your doctor to use certain pools. Many FMS patients have found the aqua jogger belt to be a fun aerobic alternative. The Arthritis Foundation has a list of warm water pools in your local area. Contact your local chapter for this information.

▲ A good book for stretching exercises is *Stretching* by Bob Anderson. ($9.95) This can be purchased in bookstores, or your local library might carry a copy for you to check out.

▲ The Arthritis Foundation offers exercise classes in many communities. You can call them for specifics. They offer a warm water exercise program designed for people with arthritis that might be good to try.

▲ Remember to be flexible in your exercise program. Adjust your level to avoid over-exertion. Do not exercise if you have the flu or are feeling bad. Skip a day and then start again the next.

▲ In some health clubs there are people knowledgeable of FMS who can help guide you in an exercise program. However, some health club personnel do not understand that "no pain, no gain" does not work with the FMS patient. If you find your health club personnel or physical therapist is pushing you too hard, you will need to reassess your program. Only you know how you feel!

▲ *Fibromyalgia Exercise Videos* - A good one to try is by Patty Bourne, a kinesiologist who developed a 30-minute upbeat exercise videotape for FMS patients. Sharon Clark, Ph.D., has developed a stretching exercise video which many people enjoy and is in the process of completing a strengthening video. Ordering information for the videos is included in the resource section of this book.

▲ Some FMS patients like using a Nordic Track at low levels. Many patients find they are most successful with the Nordic Track by starting only with their legs and gradually adding their arms.

▲ Do not give up!

"If you constantly think and talk about your pain then you are living with it—you are never apart from it. Just as your thoughts can influence your feelings and behavior, so can your behavior influence your thoughts and feelings. If you try to act normal in everyday living as much as you can, then you will find yourself gradually less involved with your pain and less aware of it." Richard Sternbach, M.D., from *Mastering Pain: A Twelve-Step Program for Coping with Chronic Pain.*

Exercise Diary

Date	Stretching	Exercise time	How did you feel after?

Sample of Stretches

The following are a sample of stretches that are often recommended for those with fibromyalgia. It may be helpful to take a hot shower or bath before stretching. Remember to stretch gently and to hold each stretch for about ten seconds or longer, then relax. Never force a stretch; you will only experience more pain. Daily stretching can be a very beneficial component of treatment, but when it's done incorrectly, it can actually do more harm than good. Bob Anderson's book *Stretching* provides excellent stretching guidelines and has numerous illustrations which are helpful when learning specific stretches. A physical therapist can individualize a stretching program for you and help ensure that you are stretching both correctly and safely. Remember that accurate information on stretching and individual guidance form the foundation for a good stretching program.

Important Note

Please consult your physician before you begin a stretching program. Some individuals with FMS have complicating physical problems that can be aggravated by stretching—a situation which you certainly would want to avoid!

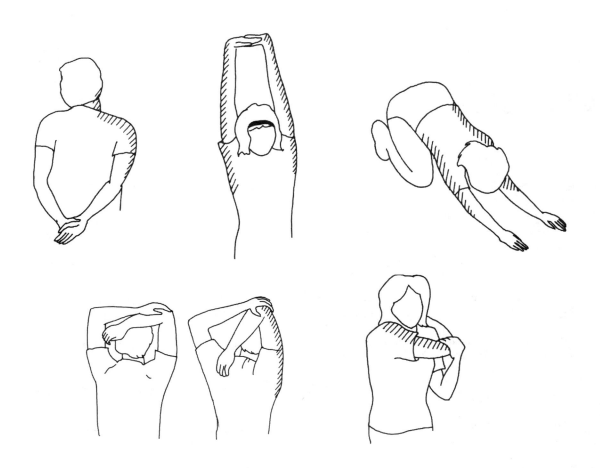

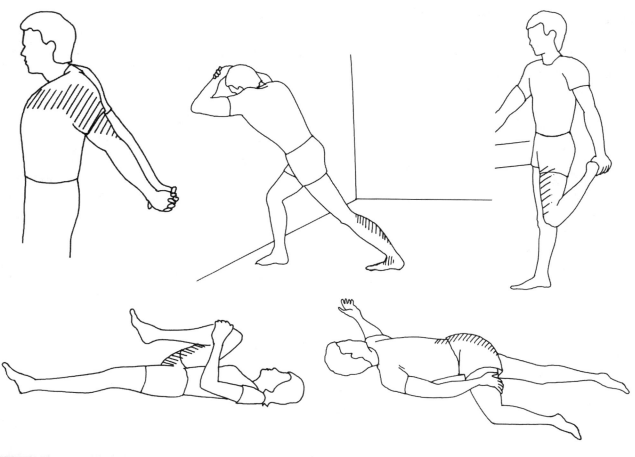

REFERENCES

Anderson, Bob. *Stretching.* Bolinas, CA: Shelter Publications, Inc., 1980.

Bennett, R.M., et al. Aerobic fitness in patients with fibrositis. *Arthritis and Rheum,* 32, (4), 454-460, 1989.

Cardahl, K. Dyspnea in chronic primary fibromyalgia. *J. Intern Med,* 226, (4), 265-270, 1989.

Clark, S.R., Burckhardt, C.S., Bennett, R.M. FM patients improve oxygen consumption and pain score during a 3 month program of aerobic exercise, *J Musculoskeletal Pain,* 3(1):70, 1995.

Gowans, Susan, Voss, Susan, deHueck, Amy, Richardson, Mary. A Randomized Controlled Trial of Exercise and Education in Fibromyalgia. 387. Scientific Abstracts. ACR Annual Meeting. October, 1996.

Jacobsen, S., Danneskiold-Sams. Dynamic muscular endurance in primary fibromyalgia compared with chronic myofascial pain syndrome. *Archives of Physical Medicine and Rehabilitation,* 73 (2), 170-173, 1992.

Kazyama, H.H.S., et al. Fibromyalgia: Continuous physical therapy program with or without long term medical supervision, *Journal of Musculoskeletal Pain,* 3(1):126, 1995.

McCain, Glenn. A controlled study of the effects of a supervised cardiovascular fitness training program on the manifestations of primary fibromyalgia. *Arth Rheum,* 31, (9), 1135-1141, 1988.

Mengshoel, A.M., Höllestad, N.K., Förre, O. Pain and fatigue induced by exercise in fibromyalgia patients and sedentary health subjects, *Clinical and Experimental Rheumatology,* 13:477-482, 1995.

Novregaard, J., et al. Exercise training in treatment of fibromyalgia, *J Musculoskeletal Pain,* 3(1):105, 1995.

Sternbach, Richard. *Mastering Pain: A Twelve-Step Program for Coping with Chronic Pain.* New York: Ballantine, 1987.

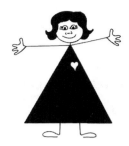

Doctor/Patient Relationship

The relationship that you have with your doctor can certainly influence the success you will have in learning to manage your symptoms of FMS. A positive relationship embraces good communication and listening skills and relies on accurate, timely information to be provided by both parties. Important components of good communication within the doctor/patient relationship are the following.

    ▲ **Have reasonable expectations**

    ▲ **Exchange concise, accurate information**

    ▲ **Exercise good listening skills**

    ▲ **Ask questions of each other**

    ▲ **Be willing to express feelings and concerns**

The rewards and benefits of developing good communication between you and your doctor can be mutual respect and trust of one another. These are certainly attributes that will help empower you to take charge of your fibromyalgia.

Within this relationship, you have rights and responsibilities that are important to recognize and become committed to in order to receive well-coordinated health care that meets your individual needs.

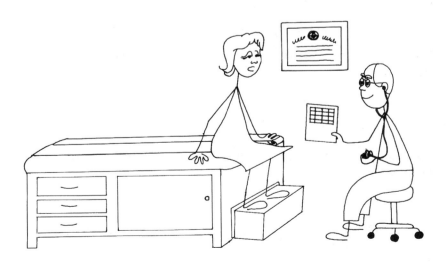

Patient Rights

- ▲ To have your needs and concerns listened to
- ▲ To be recognized and respected as an individual
- ▲ To receive quality medical care
- ▲ To be involved in the medical decisions that affect your life
- ▲ To ask for help and support
- ▲ To be informed and educated

Patient Responsibilities

- ▲ Provide concise, accurate information (e.g., medical history, current symptoms, sleep quality, current and past medications).
- ▲ Accurately report adverse fibromyalgia symptoms and side effects of medications.
- ▲ Become educated. (This will help enable you to ask the appropriate questions, form reasonable expectations, and recognize what information is important to record and report.)
- ▲ Be an active participant in your treatment. (Listen, ask questions, give feedback, follow through with treatment to the best of your ability.)
- ▲ Be honest in expressing feelings and concerns.

Office Visit

- ▲ Be concise and well organized.
- ▲ Ask your most important questions at the beginning of the visit.
- ▲ Summarize information which will help your doctor assess your particular situation.
- ▲ Discuss types of treatment that you feel may be helpful.
- ▲ Develop a flare-up plan.
- ▲ Ask for clarification if you are unclear about any part of your treatment or medical care.

When preparing for your office visit, remember that you will need to be concise and well organized in order to discuss your needs and concerns with your doctor in a short period of time. Our changing health care environment with its myriad of insurance restrictions is putting increased demands on our physicians and often limitations on the standard office visit. As a patient, you must strive to make good use of your allotted time and focus on those issues or questions that must be addressed by your physician.

Identify your three most important questions and/or concerns and be sure to ask them at the beginning of your visit. When choosing the questions to ask your doctor, review your list and consider who is the most appropriate health professional to answer each question. You may have questions on your list that would be best answered by your physical therapist, dietician, pharmacist, nurse clinician, etc., which would then leave more time in the office visit for those concerns most appropriate for your physician. If your doctor doesn't attempt to answer your questions, let him/her know how important it is that you have time to discuss these concerns at this visit. If your situation is unusually complex and you have a number of concerns that cannot be addressed in a standard office visit, ask the individual who schedules the appointments how he/she would prefer to handle this situation.

To help your doctor better assess your particular situation, it's often helpful to bring a summary of concise, accurate information to your office visit. For example, if you've been having difficulty sleeping in recent weeks, summarize your sleep patterns over the past several weeks and list the medications that you've been taking during this time with their specific dosages. If your symptoms have increased, be prepared to describe them.

If there are various types of treatment that you feel may be helpful to you in better managing your fibromyalgia, discuss them briefly with your doctor. Examples might be biofeedback training, counseling, physical therapy, warm water pool exercise, etc. If he/she feels that you would benefit from a particular treatment, remember to obtain a prescription if necessary before leaving your appointment. It's also helpful to know what types of treatment are covered by your insurance and, in some cases, how many visits you are allowed.

Some individuals have found it beneficial to develop a plan with their physician that could be easily implemented when they have a flare-up of their symptoms. This plan will certainly vary from doctor to doctor and patient to patient, but may include several sessions of physical therapy, a small increase in medication or addition of another medication, massage, etc. Some physicians will prefer to be notified of a flare-up that is difficult to manage and will individually assess the situation and make specific recommendations. Do not make any adjustments in your medication(s) without first discussing dosage options with your physician.

As you are coming to the end of your office visit, ask for clarification if you are unclear about any part of your treatment or medical care. You may benefit from taking brief notes during your visit and/or repeating back to your doctor, in your own words, what you understand him/her to have said.

The following questions have been designed to help you narrow the focus of your office visit and assist you in getting the most out of a short period of time. We encourage you to read through the questions and use them to organize your thoughts before your next appointment.

The patient can provide invaluable information to his/her doctor which will be used for diagnosis and subsequent treatment. Before your visit, ask yourself:

▲ What is the main reason that I'm going to the doctor today?

▲ What are the three most important questions that I would like to ask my doctor? (Write these down and take to appointment.)

▲ What else worries me about my health?

▲ What do I expect the doctor to do for me today?

During the office visit, ask your doctor any or all of the following (as appropriate):

▲ What tests will need to be done?

▲ What is your diagnosis? (Ask doctor to write it down if necessary.)

▲ Medications? What? When? For how long? Possible concerns or side effects?

▲ Is there any treatment that could be helpful? What? Activity? Precautions?

▲ Are there any helpful patient education materials available for the condition?

▲ Any other recommendations?

At the end of the visit, ask your doctor any or all of the following (as appropriate):

▲ Am I to return for another visit? Yes/No? When?

▲ Should I report back to you by telephone for any reason? Yes/No? When?

▲ What symptoms and/or side effects from treatment or medications do you want to be informed of?

▲ Am I to call in for test results? Yes/No? When?

▲ If a problem arises with medication or treatment, may I call for an answer rather than make another appointment?

Phone Calls

If you're experiencing side effects from a medication and/or problems with a specific treatment, call your physician for advice. Adjustments in medication and/or treatments can usually be briefly discussed on the phone and will help you avoid undue suffering.

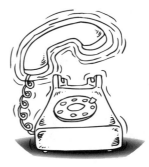

▲ Don't expect your doctor to remember the details of your particular situation.

▲ Describe the problem or ask the question that concerns you the most at the beginning of the conversation.
Example: It is often helpful to write down the specifics you wish to cover and put them by your phone.

- Be specific and concise.
  Example: If your question concerns your sleep and medication, know approximately how many times that you've been waking at night and the range of total hours that you've been sleeping. Also have a list of your current medication(s) with specific dosage(s) by the phone.

- Have the phone number of your pharmacy handy in case your doctor wants to phone in a prescription for you.

- Be prepared to jot down any medical advice that you're given.
  Example: How long should you expect to take a new medication before noticing some improvement in your sleep quality?

- Ask your doctor when he/she wants to be contacted and/or when you should come in for an office visit.

The memory and concentration problems that are common in many individuals with fibromyalgia often contribute to poorly organized and incomplete phone conversations. The work that you do in preparing for a phone call and the notes that you take during the call will help you obtain the information you need and also help assure that you will remember the important details.

Nurture a healthy, positive doctor/patient relationship; the benefits are many. As a patient, educate yourself so that you will know best what questions to ask and how to be proactive in your medical care. Take the responsibility of reporting to your physician undue side effects of medications, increased sleep disruptions, a flare-up of symptoms that doesn't respond to your efforts and other issues that concern you. A physician who is sensitive to your needs can help empower you to manage your symptoms from day to day and can use creative problem-solving and management skills in coordinating an individual plan of care for you. Conversely, a physician who is not willing to work with you and provide guidance in the management of your fibromyalgia can actually contribute to the frustrations and challenges that you may already be experiencing. If you decide that you need to see a different physician, ask a leader of a local FMS support group for recommendations of physicians who are knowledgeable about FMS and who work well with FMS patients. A local arthritis care center may also be a resource for physicians.

"The quality of the doctor/patient relationship can mean the difference between a well-managed illness and needless wasted time and aggravation. Being assertive, believing in yourself, having confidence and possessing knowledge about your condition will help you enlist your doctor's cooperation and enhance your likelihood of successful treatment." (Rebekah Milaro, FMS patient and contributing writer to *Fibromyalgia Network*, October 1991)

Doctor/Patient Resource

Book: *Examining Your Doctor*

An excellent resource on evaluating the quality of your medical care is *Examining Your Doctor* by Timothy McCall, M.D. Cost: $16.95 + 4.00 shipping and handling in the U.S. and $23.95 in Canada. Carol Publishing Group, 120 Enterprise Avenue, Secaucus, NJ 07094 (800) 447-2665.

Disrespectful Medical Treatment

Jenny Fransen, R.N.

Only recently has medical science begun to understand the underlying mechanism for fibromyalgia. For many years it was not well understood; consequently, many people with this disorder spent years searching for a diagnosis and effective treatment to relieve their pain. The average length of time from onset of symptoms to diagnosis has been approximately eight years. Unfortunately, during this pre-diagnosis period, many people have met with countless health care professionals who were insensitive, disrespectful, uneducated, and who blamed the patient for their pain. They were told they were crazy, "It's all in your head," and other damaging comments.

If you have had this experience, it is important for you to know you are not to blame for your symptoms. You are not crazy. You have a real medical condition, and you deserve respectful medical treatment. The damaging comments that were directed toward you were completely inappropriate. You have a right to be angry about this mistreatment.

It is also important for you to know that receiving this type of treatment over a prolonged period of time may cause you to distrust and feel angry toward all medical professionals. This anger and distrust, if left unchecked, can interfere in new relationships with health care professionals and refuel the cycle to be repeated.

Guilt and shame are also painful emotions felt by many people with fibromyalgia as a response to disrespect and blame by medical professionals. They are the feelings "I must be bad because I have this," or "I must somehow be at fault for having this." These feelings can lead to depression if they are prolonged and left unchecked. They can negatively impact one's adjustment to living with this medical condition.

Isolation is another painful experience people with fibromyalgia can experience, as a result of not receiving the understanding needed to live with chronic muscle pain and fatigue. It is the result of not feeling like there is anyone available who believes and understands what you are living with day after day. Feelings of isolation and loneliness are also extremely common because fibromyalgia is invisible to the naked eye. No one around you can see or feel your pain.

It is important to take some time to evaluate who has given you disrespectful care in the past, and what responses you have developed as a result of mistreatment. It might be helpful to make a list.

How can you express your anger toward those who have hurt you? You could write them a letter and express how their treatment hurt you, how you now have received a correct diagnosis, and what they could have done which would have been more helpful. Some people choose to send the letter, and others do not. It can help to put some closure on the relationship, as well as help you to diffuse some of the anger toward the ones who have caused the pain. You may want to send information to educate them on fibromyalgia so they don't continue to hurt others with this condition. However you choose to deal with your anger, it's important to focus it constructively towards those who hurt you, not toward anyone else. Continuing to feel anger for prolonged periods of time hurts you. Find constructive outlets to ventilate your anger. Try writing in a journal. Find people with whom you can talk about it. Anger is an energy that can be used constructively to motivate you to help yourself feel better, to help other people, and to be proactive as a health care consumer and in your program of self-care.

Lastly, you must not remain under disrespectful medical care. It will only continue to harm your sense of well-being, fuel depression and anger, and continue the cycle of distrust toward medical professionals. You must find respectful, caring medical professionals who believe you and do not blame you for your pain. You deserve respectful care, and you must have it.

Seek out an understanding person or counselor to help you resolve any painful experiences or emotions. By getting support, you can work through your experience so it doesn't continue to hurt you as deeply. Getting support can also help to reduce the isolation and depression that you may be experiencing. Remember to elicit support from those people who believe you and who are understanding.

▲▲▲

TIPS Working with Your Physician

Jenny Fransen, R.N.

▲ Prepare for the visit ahead of time to make the best use of your short time together.

▲ Be sensitive to your own symptoms and concerns and give some thought to the questions that you might ask your doctor.

▲ Keep a list handy to jot questions down between office visits.

▲ Consider other resources for information, such as your pharmacist for medication questions.

▲ As there is no magic bullet for fibromyalgia, great patience is required to find a combination of therapies and medication to bring about improvement.

▲ Recognize that there will be inherent frustrations for patients and physicians when treating a condition that continues to hold many mysteries for the researchers.

▲ Realize much of your treatment is up to you: exercise, relaxation, stress management, pain management, pursuing additional therapies and treatments such as biofeedback, spray and stretch, and massage.

▲ Learn as much as you can about your own disease, since you are the one who will manage the day-to-day problems that occur.

▲ Actively manage fibromyalgia-related problems, such as pain, sleep problems, etc.

▲ During office visits be prepared to ask for what you need to manage your fibromyalgia. Be as specific and as concise as possible. Don't ramble.

▲ Work with your physician to develop a plan of action should you have a flare-up so you can initiate treatment on your own. Can you increase your sleep medication or take ibuprofen for pain? What else can you do during a flare-up to reduce symptoms and feel better?

▲ If you are having symptoms of depression, inform your physician. Depression can further disrupt sleep cycles and will need treatment.

DOCTOR/PATIENT

▲ Reinforce and thank the doctor for specific behaviors and techniques you find helpful. "I appreciate that you really listen to me, Dr. Olson."

▲ Learn to ask for what you need from your physician. "Would you explain to me what can be done to help me sleep better?"

▲ Develop a good relationship with the doctor's nurse and receptionist. Identify rules of the office: doctor's day off and when the best time is to call and leave a message. Know the nurse's name and ask for him/her when you call. Be patient if they are unable to call back immediately.

▲ Identify any bad feelings you might have about delayed diagnosis, insensitive treatment, etc. Resolve these if possible with the appropriate person in person or by letter. In this way, you avoid carrying bad feelings toward health care providers into future relationships.

▲ Should you and your physician have difficulties, try to identify problems and work to resolve them. You can put your feelings into a letter if you aren't able to express them in person.

▲ Avoid angry or defensive communication.

▲ If your physician has told you to return in three months, you can make an appointment earlier to discuss your questions or concerns if necessary.

▲ If a problem arises with medication or treatment, ask if you can call for an answer rather than make another appointment.

▲ Be assertive and take responsibility for your own treatment.

▲ Remember **you** are in charge of your own treatment program.

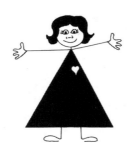

Work-Related Issues

Fibromyalgia may affect a person's ability to perform on the job. The symptoms of chronic pain and fatigue and difficulties with memory and concentration can be especially challenging for some people. 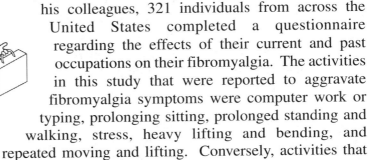 It's also recognized that certain work tasks or types of employment can potentially aggravate fibromyalgia symptoms. In a study by G.W. Waylonis, M.D., and his colleagues, 321 individuals from across the United States completed a questionnaire regarding the effects of their current and past occupations on their fibromyalgia. The activities in this study that were reported to aggravate fibromyalgia symptoms were computer work or typing, prolonging sitting, prolonged standing and walking, stress, heavy lifting and bending, and repeated moving and lifting. Conversely, activities that did not appear to exacerbate the symptoms of fibromyalgia included walking, variable light sedentary work, teaching, light desk work, and phone work. In conclusion, light sedentary occupations that allow for varied tasks and changing positions appeared to be tolerated the best.

For many, it is worthwhile to spend time identifying potential problem areas in your job and then to begin identifying possible solutions. For example:

▲ Are you engaged in prolonged repetitive activities?
Could you take frequent short breaks to stretch, relax and/or do some biofeedback?

▲ Are you in one position for sustained periods of time?
Changing positions frequently, if only for a few minutes, could be helpful.

▲ Is your neck, shoulder and/or back pain aggravated by postural strain? Check the position of your work surface, chair, computer, etc., to determine if they are at the proper heights to help you maintain good posture.

▲ Are you in a job with high stress?
Would it be possible to take short breaks to relax, do some abdominal breathing, practice biofeedback, stretch, etc.? Are there tasks that could be delegated? Could you take a stress management class to learn a variety of ways to better manage stress?

Be creative in identifying potential solutions, try several, and then further adapt them to your situation. An occupational therapist may assist you in assessing your specific needs and then make various recommendations to you and to your employer. You might also ask yourself the following questions:

▲ How could I do my job differently?

▲ How could I rearrange or modify the way various tasks are done?

▲ How might I pace myself and my work tasks better throughout the day?

▲ Could I adjust my work schedule or discuss the option of flexible working hours with my employer?

▲ Could I decrease my hours and work part-time?

Continue to explore all of the options and make the necessary changes or adjustments that will help you better manage your FMS within your work environment. Your employer may be more willing to work with you in making these accommodations if you ask your physician to write a letter describing your symptoms of fibromyalgia and explaining your specific limitations. Any suggestions that he/she could include regarding changes or accommodations that would likely be helpful for you would help underscore your requests.

The Americans with Disabilities Act (ADA) requires employers to make reasonable adjustments and accommodations for people with disabilities and chronic illnesses. The ADA was amended in 1994 to exempt companies with fewer than 15 employees, while requiring those companies with 15 or more employees to follow the guidelines. You might consider asking your employer what resources and support services are available to help evaluate your specific needs and make recommendations for you. For more information on the Americans with Disabilities Act contact: U.S. Equal Employment Opportunity Commission, Publication and Information Center, P.O. Box 12549, Cincinnati, Ohio 45212-0549 (800) 669-3362.

Some individuals with fibromyalgia may continue to have a lot of difficulty in their jobs even after making a variety of changes and accommodations. Some may feel that they're unable to work in their current position, at least for a time. If you find that you are unable to perform your job, discuss this situation with your physician. Also find out what other options are available to you at work. You may need to take a leave of absence from your current position and use that time to become more involved in a variety of treatments for your fibromyalgia, with a goal of better managing your symptoms and returning to work. You may also choose to explore other job options during this time and/or programs for retraining or vocational counseling. Check into whether you have short-term or long-term disability insurance benefits available through your job or through an independent insurance policy. Those individuals who were injured on the job may be able to receive Worker's Compensation benefits for medical expenses, retraining and/or lost income.

If you have been off of work or have been working part-time due to your fibromyalgia symptoms, it may be beneficial for you to consider gradually returning to work. Start with a minimum of hours that you feel you can work and then slowly increase your work hours over the following weeks and months. Try to avoid overtime and shift work if possible; the latter may be particularly troublesome. If you have the option, work a variety of days and times and vary the number of hours worked per day. See what works best for you! Continue to increase your hours while assessing your ability to function in your job and manage your fibromyalgia. If you experience increased symptoms that aren't tolerable as you work more hours, you may need to reduce your work schedule again for a time. Charting your progress in a journal could help you make wise employment decisions. Remember to work closely with both your physician and employer during these times of transition.

Although many people with fibromyalgia continue to be employed, there are individuals with this condition who find that they are unable to do any kind of work despite a variety of attempts to do so. An option for these people is to apply for Social Security disability. This can be a difficult process for many because claim administrators often don't have a good understanding of fibromyalgia, and sometimes patients will find that their own physician is less than willing to write a letter for them in support of disability.

Attorneys experienced in fibromyalgia disability claims may provide invaluable assistance with the necessary paperwork, hearings, etc. They will also be familiar with the components that often increase the likelihood of a successful claim for disability. If you need help in locating an attorney familiar with fibromyalgia, contact your state or local bar association for assistance. Members of a local support group may also be familiar with attorneys who are knowledgeable and experienced in fibromyalgia disability claims.

The work status and prevalence of disability in people with fibromyalgia has been studied by Frederick Wolfe, M.D., and colleagues. In a survey of 1668 FMS patients from seven centers with diverse socio-economic characteristics, they found that 65.4% reported being able to work most or all days, while 18.9% stated they could work few or no days. When assessing all disability sources, these investigators found that 25.3% of the patients had received a disability payment, while 74.7% reported that they had never received a disability award. In this same study, almost 15% of patients had received Social Security Disability (SSD) payments, compared to 2.2% of the total U.S. population (U.S. Social Security Administration data). In an attempt to understand the reason for the SSD awards, a small subgroup of 52 patients who had received Social Security disability were surveyed. Twenty-three percent reported an award specifically for fibromyalgia, 19.2% for "arthritis," 23.1% for back problems or miscellaneous musculoskeletal problems, 1.9% for systemic lupus erythematosus, 9.7% for psychiatric reasons, 17.3% for non-rheumatic medical reasons and 3.9% for unknown reasons.

While we know that fibromyalgia may affect your ability to perform on the job, we encourage you to explore a variety of options that potentially may help you better manage your FMS within your work environment. Remember to be creative in identifying the possible changes, solutions and/or adaptations that might be beneficial to you. Many of you will find that as you implement some of these changes and adjust them specifically to your work scenario, managing fibromyalgia and work can be a successful venture.

REFERENCES

Henriksson, C., Burckhardt, C. Impact of fibromyalgia on everyday life: a study of women in the USA and Sweden. *Disability and Rehabilitation*, 18(5):241-8, May 1996.

Waylonis, G.W., Ronan, P.G. and Gordon, C. A profile of fibromyalgia in occupational environments. *American Journal of Physical Medicine and Rehabilitation*, 73(2):112-5, April 1994.

Wolfe, F., Anderson, J., Harkness, D., Bennett, R.M., Caro, X., Goldenberg, D.M., Russell, I.J. and Yunus, M.B. The Work and Disability Status of Persons with Fibromyalgia. Abstract presented at 1995 ACR/ARHP Annual Meeting, October 1995.

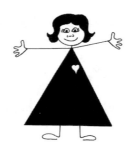

Stress Management/Relaxation

Stress is not an external event that produces anxiety or frustration in our bodies; it is our own physical and emotional reaction to external events taking place around us and within us. Studies have shown that there are actual physical changes occurring in our bodies when we are stressed.

Changes which can occur are:

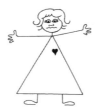

- ▲ Muscle tension and pain
- ▲ Stomach distress
- ▲ Headaches
- ▲ Heart irregularities
- ▲ Anxiety
- ▲ Depression

- ▲ Teeth grinding/TMJ
- ▲ High blood pressure
- ▲ Cold hands/feet
- ▲ Insomnia
- ▲ Ulcers
- ▲ Diarrhea/constipation

Chronic stress can deplete the body of many chemicals needed for proper functioning, and we can develop various diseases as a result. Research also shows that we can take steps to change the way we respond to stress and create a healing atmosphere for our bodies. Each person needs to identify the major stressors in his or her life, realize how they are affecting him or her psychologically and/or physically, and, above all, what methods to use to alleviate stress.

One of the reasons fibromyalgia can be such a difficult thing to live with is because of its unpredictability. This in itself is very stressful. If only someone could tell you how you are going to feel in six months, or one year or ten years from now, it would at least alleviate some of the uncertainty of living with an illness whose symptoms catch us by surprise day to day, week to week, or even hour to hour! We constantly wonder what we did wrong to cause our flare or what we did right to alleviate our symptoms. Our days, weeks and months are up and down, like a roller coaster, and we are hanging on for dear life, wondering when the next flare will send us racing head first to the bottom of the roller coaster. We need to learn to deal with the physical stresses of that ride, as well as the emotional stressors. People who have an easier time accepting this uncertainty seem to do better overall than those people who cannot handle the flares and remissions of FMS. Other people (the lucky ones) who have a milder form of FMS find that the ups and downs are less severe and less frequent, therefore less stressful. Others say that just as they manage to have a good spell, FMS ambushes them again and they find it difficult to control all the emotional and painful effects of this new attack. This pattern is not easy to cope with, but you need to learn how to handle these flares both physically and emotionally for them to be less stressful. Accepting the fact that flares will happen and are part of the illness can be a healthy step toward dealing with the ups and downs of living with FMS.

Chronic Stress Can Lead to Severe Illness: Chronic Illness Is Severely Stressing

Everyone with fibromyalgia agrees that stress aggravates their symptoms. As fibromyalgia patients, we must identify what our own stressors are and learn how to cope with them to enhance our self-esteem as well as reduce our painful symptoms.

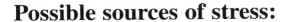

Everyone reacts differently to stress. What is perceived as stressful to one person may be unnoticed by another. It is necessary for you to locate the sources of your own personal stress factors so you can reduce them or learn effective ways of coping or controlling them. It is not always the big things in life that create stress for us, but oftentimes stress can be caused by the little things that pile up on a day-to-day basis and send our nervous system into overload.

Possible sources of stress:

▲ Marital relations
▲ Work
▲ Friends
▲ Lack of support system
▲ Guilt
▲ Loneliness
▲ Depression
▲ Sexual difficulties
▲ Inadequate nutrition
▲ Commitments

▲ Everyday hassles
▲ Finances
▲ Hurriedness
▲ Perfectionism
▲ Anger
▲ FMS
▲ Anxiety
▲ Holidays
▲ Alcohol, nicotine & caffeine
▲ Worry

Reduce, Eliminate, Negotiate: Balance Is Necessary to Reduce Stress

Look over your life for possible stressors–check this list and mark any that affect you. You might even have more to add! These can all aggravate your fibromyalgia. Try to rid yourself of toxic friends, too many committee meetings, or a job that is giving you little satisfaction and aggravates your fibromyalgia symptoms. Learn to let go of guilt, anger, perfectionism, hurriedness, and obsessive-compulsive behavior. This is easier said than done! Some people may need professional help in overcoming self-defeating behaviors. Social workers, therapists or psychiatrists might be helpful in sorting out these problems. Finding a qualified therapist who relates well with you is important. Anxiety and depression may decrease, as well as some of your fibromyalgia symptoms. Work out problems with your boss or in-laws–you will feel better. Talk to your children and spouse about your fibromyalgia and ask for help and their support. Above all, surround yourself with supportive people, who will likely include various members of your family, circle of friends and health care team. Set aside 20 minutes each day for "worry time." Write down all your worries so you don't have to think about them when you are in bed. This is also a good time to make a list of things you need to do the next day.

There is evidence that everyday hassles are just as stressful–if not more so–than major events. Try to simplify your living space, as well as your life. Throw out, organize, unclutter, redefine, simplify, simplify, simplify. Get psychological counseling if you can afford it. If the stressors are reduced in your life, your body can take time to heal. This might be a difficult task for some of you, but well worth the effort. There are many books available in the library on stress management, as well as community educational classes or therapists who can help you reduce stress and cope more effectively. Try to achieve a balance in your life. If your life is balanced, your body can become balanced. Renowned psychologist C.J. Jung noted that primitive people interpreted illness not as a negative, but as the unconscious coming forth to transform a person into someone better. Use this illness as a time to transform your life! Take charge of your fibromyalgia and your life!

Cognitive Behavioral Therapy
Self-Talk: What we say to ourselves affects how we feel

Researchers trying to help people with fibromyalgia have turned to Cognitive Behavioral Therapy as an additional method of alleviating painful symptoms. A therapist using this technique would teach you how to control disturbing emotional reactions by suggesting more effective ways of interpreting and thinking about your experiences. For example, if you make a mistake at work you might say to yourself, "I am the most stupid person in the world! I always make mistakes!" The therapist would point out that you do not always make mistakes and that everyone makes mistakes and feels foolish at one time or another. The behavioral aspect of this therapy would have you noting your mood or feelings when you are thinking these thoughts. Painful emotions such as guilt, shame, and anxiety can aggravate pain and your fibromyalgia. We are our thoughts. Negative thinking produces negative behavior. Some research suggests negative thinking causes illness. If negative thinking causes illness, can positive thinking create health? There are many researchers who believe this is possible. If this idea sounds foolish to you, and you decide it would never benefit your fibromyalgia symptoms, you are probably feeling skeptical and discouraged or maybe even angry. Your pain level may increase as you are having these thoughts. On the other hand, if this sounds like a great idea to you, you may feel an uplift in your mood. If you pay attention to your body at the same time, you may notice a slight decrease in your pain level. Our bodies react immediately to our emotions. If we can control our thoughts, maybe we can control our bodies.

There are therapists who teach people how to change distorted or faulty thinking. If you can't afford psychotherapy, you could read *Feeling Good, the New Mood Therapy,* by David D. Burns, M.D., or his handbook, *The Feeling Good Handbook.* Some of the basic ideas of Cognitive

Behavioral Therapy are provided for you on the next page. We cannot teach this technique to you in the limited confines of this book, but we want you to have an idea of what it is all about so you can decide if it is something you should pursue.

Notice when your thoughts follow any of these patterns:

▲ **All or nothing thinking.** "I have fibromyalgia, therefore, I can't lead a normal life." Wrong. It would be better to say to yourself, "Many people lead normal lives once they get their fibromyalgia under control, and I can too."

▲ **Overgeneralization**. You see a single negative event as a never-ending pattern of defeat. "My doctor misdiagnosed me, therefore, I can never get better."

▲ **Disqualifying the positive.** Rejecting positive experiences as short-lived and possibly not recurring. "My fibromyalgia symptoms were better this weekend when I rested, but it will never happen again."

▲ **Catastrophizing.** You exaggerate the importance of things. "I can't keep my house as clean as I used to, therefore, I am a failure." Are you a failure? No, you just cannot do as much as you used to. Ask for help. Learn to live with a messier house!

▲ **Should statements.** "I should be able to do all that I did before I had fibromyalgia." You can't, and if you try, you will have a flare and frustrate yourself. Be kind to yourself. Treat yourself gently.

▲ **Personalization.** You see yourself as the cause of some negative event for which you were not responsible. "My fibromyalgia must have started because I was not taking care of myself." No one knows why fibromyalgia starts; you are not the cause of it.

When you have these problems with distorted thinking, your body reacts to your thoughts within milliseconds. Cognitive behavior therapy attempts to change your irrational thought patterns by finding the positive in your negative thinking, stopping self-blame, defusing anger, feeling overwhelmed, etc. Try to change these thought patterns. Find the positive in every negative thought you have. "I am in pain now, and will be forever." Is that true? Aren't there times when you are free of pain? If you have small amounts of time when you are free from pain, you can increase that time gradually until you have more time when you are pain-free. Notice how high your pain level is when you are thinking about your pain or when someone has made you angry or you are hurrying to get tasks accomplished. Notice how low your pain level is when you are relaxed or in a hot bath. Researchers feel that psychological factors can influence the degree of pain we feel. It has been found that people with fibromyalgia have significantly more negative feelings about themselves, more pain preoccupation, less support from significant others, more psychosomatic symptoms, less job satisfaction and poorer future expectations than patients with rheumatoid arthritis. If you can develop healthier attitudes, change negative thinking, and be optimistic, your fibromyalgia symptoms can and will decrease. It might take many months to have a beneficial effect if you attempt to change your thought patterns, but it is worth trying. You have nothing to lose and everything to gain.

One other technique which is easy to implement is to use positive affirmations throughout the day. We have provided a list of some for you to try. It is better to say these out loud and repeat them on a consistent basis for the affirmations to work. Try repeating to yourself as you exercise or do your daily stretches: "Every day in every way, I am getting better and better." Repeat it ten times three or four times a day, every day for a month. See if it helps you.   Some people find it helpful to write down positive affirmations on a card and carry it in their purse or pocket. Reading the card a few times during the day can help keep your positive thoughts on track whenever negative thinking creeps into your mind.

Positive Thoughts for Coping with Fibromyalgia

▲   I am confident of my ability to deal with my health and live a good life.

▲   Things are getting better.

▲   I am making progress in helping myself to feel better.

▲   Today I can do what I need to do for my recovery.

▲   I can treat myself gently and with the special care I would give a close friend.

▲   I am learning what I need to do to take care of my body.

▲   I focus on positive actions I can take to advocate for myself.

▲   I look for the good this day can bring.

▲   I go with the flow of each new day accepting what I can learn from it.

▲   I seek out the positive support I need to live with fibromyalgia.

▲   I let go of any muscle tension or problems over which I have no control.

▲   I live with positive expectancy: each day I expect to feel better and more relaxed.

▲   I counter each stress with techniques I know to balance out negative stress.

▲   I can surmount any problem that occurs today with calm problem-solving skills.

▲   I can look for the resources I need to manage any problems.

▲   I maintain slow and easy breathing bringing fresh oxygen to my muscles and breathe out muscle waste products.

▲   I keep my muscles loose and relaxed throughout the day.

▲   I take time during the day to relax and breathe to refresh my muscles.

▲   I creatively manage the problems each new day brings.

▲   I can do whatever I need to do to take good care of myself.

Relaxation Techniques

Relaxation techniques are another useful adjunct to stress management. By relaxation we do not mean the relaxing you do in front of the television with your family at night, although this has its place in reducing stress as well. The relaxation techniques we refer to are those that banish tension from our bodies as well as our minds. Some of these techniques are being used by doctors for their fibromyalgia patients as an addition to their overall treatment plan. Studies show that those people who practice these techniques regularly have had significant reductions in their pain levels and an increase in their sense of well-being. Many fibromyalgia patients complain that they can't relax their muscles. This can be learned through the regular practice of these techniques.

There are many advantages to learning these techniques. Relaxation produces the opposite effect on our bodies that stress does. Relaxation

- **Lowers heart rate, blood pressure and oxygen consumption**

- **Reduces blood lactate level, which is a chemical produced in large quantities when we are faced with stress**

- **Produces brain EEG wave changes that are of benefit**

- **Increases production of serotonin**

- **Is psychologically and physiologically more refreshing and energy restoring than deep sleep**

Various relaxation techniques include

- **Meditation**
- **Relaxation tapes**
- **Hypnosis**

- **Yoga**
- **Biofeedback**
- **Tai Chi**

You should choose the one most suited to your personality.

Basic Rules for Relaxation

- They must be practiced regularly to be effective. Five or six times a week for 20 to 40 minutes is a target to aim for.

- You will need a quiet room, free of distraction. (Sometimes this is hard to find.)

- Wear loose, comfortable clothing.

- Practice diaphragmatic breathing the entire time you practice relaxing.

- Anyone can learn to do this–it's like learning to ride a bicycle!

- When you first start practicing, you may find it difficult to stay still for that long. Don't try to force relaxation; it will come naturally. The more you practice the more effective it will become. Try starting with only five to ten minutes. Gradually increase the length of time as your ability to concentrate increases.

- Don't expect results for at least six to eight weeks. Dramatic improvement can occur at this time.

Abdominal/Diaphragmatic Breathing

- ▲ Smooth
- ▲ Inhalation same as exhalation
- ▲ Breathe through the nose
- ▲ Deep

- ▲ Slow
- ▲ Gentle
- ▲ Posture is straight
- ▲ Pay attention to the breath

It is impossible to be tense when you are breathing deeply. To breathe abdominally, or diaphragmatically, place your hand on your diaphragm (midway between your navel and your chest) and as you breathe feel your diaphragm expand and rise, not your chest. If your chest rises when you breathe, you are breathing too shallowly.

It is also important to pay attention throughout the day to how you are breathing. Are you holding your breath? This creates tension. Our bodies need the oxygen we breathe in for all of its functions. If you hold your breath, your body is deprived of the "breath of life"! Take time throughout the day to notice if you are breathing shallowly. If you are, take a few minutes to remind yourself to breathe from the abdomen. Breathe deeply! You will be rewarded by less tension!

Meditation

Meditation is a relaxation technique which has been around for over 2,000 years. It is simple to learn and cost-effective. All you need is a quiet room, yourself and 15 to 30 minutes. The object of meditation is to quiet the mind, emptying it of unnecessary "chatter," and achieve a state of profound harmony between body and mind.

How to meditate:

- ▲ Sit or lie down in a comfortable position in a quiet environment. Legs should be uncrossed. Wear loose comfortable clothes.

- ▲ Close your eyes.

- ▲ Breathe through your nose, practicing diaphragmatic breathing.

- ▲ Deeply relax your muscles, beginning at your feet, progressing up to your face. Pay attention to each body part until it feels relaxed and then move on to the next. Take your time so each body part has a chance to relax. Notice your toes and relax them, then your feet, ankles, calves, knees, thighs, pelvic area, abdomen, buttocks, hips, chest, arms, hands, shoulders, chest, neck, jaw, face, forehead and back.

- ▲ Become aware of your breathing after you have relaxed your entire body. Saying a one-syllable word like "one," "peace," "love," or any other word sacred and pleasing to you as you exhale is a part of the meditation technique.

- ▲ It doesn't matter what time of day you practice. You do need to be awake, so try not to fall asleep while meditating.

- ▲ Continue this for 20 to 30 minutes. Do not use an alarm to time yourself.

- ▲ When you are done, sit quietly for a few minutes. When you get up you might be amazed by how refreshed you feel.

You might find it difficult at first to concentrate only on your breathing, but that is the object. As thoughts come into your mind, be aware of them and then let them drift away. If you have a painful area, become aware of it, too. Many people find that once they pay "attention" to their pain while in a meditative state, the pain lessens. The object is not to work on a specific area; the entire body is the focus. Regular meditators have overcome addictions to tranquilizers, high blood pressure, pain, anxiety and even fibromyalgia.

Relaxation Tapes

Some people prefer using relaxation tapes to help them in their relaxation "journey." Some of these tapes include guided imagery, which transports you to a peaceful area such as a beach or garden and then guides you through images which are designed to produce muscular and mind relaxation. Many tapes have soft background music or ocean sounds which are very pleasant and calming. The person guiding you on your "journey" usually has a very soothing voice.

Some tapes are designed for specific needs such as headache relief, stress reduction, insomnia, healing, pain reduction, etc. The tapes are not expensive: the price range is between $10 and $20. You can plug these into your tape player and relax. If you have a walkman you can listen to tapes on planes, cars, at the beach or even while you wait for your next doctor's appointment. You could buy a few different tapes and have a variety to choose from. You can find them in specialty stores in your area or they can be ordered over the phone from 1-800 numbers. Some psychotherapists, nurses or hypnotherapists can tailor-make a tape for you. These, of course, would be more expensive. You can tape your own if you like. Like meditation, relaxation must be practiced daily to be effective. These tapes have also been effective for some patients who have trouble sleeping at night. If you cannot find 20 or 30 minutes in your day to listen to a tape, maybe you can find 10 minutes a day to set aside for yourself.

Hypnosis

Hypnosis is well documented as being effective in reducing anxiety and pain. Controlled studies have proven hypnotherapy effective for the treatment of some fibromyalgia symptoms. A trained hypnotherapist will guide you into a trance-like state which is very similar to deep relaxation. He or she will then guide you through a series of suggestions to reduce pain, eliminate stress and anxiety, help you sleep, etc. It is not known how hypnotism works. It just does. These sessions can be taped so you can practice at home. About 90% of the population can be hypnotized, and it is safe when done by a properly trained therapist. There usually is a society in each state for hypnotists; many are psychologists or medical doctors who use hypnotism in their practice. It would be helpful to find one who specializes in pain, relaxation, stress reduction or anxiety.

Yoga

Yoga is another relaxation technique that not only relaxes your mind, but provides stretching and flexibility for your body. There are yoga classes, books and videotapes available. You can learn the stretches and then practice them at home every day or every other day for the most benefit. Fibromyalgia patients need to stretch, and yoga provides some great stretching exercises–just remember not to strain too much. You don't want to hurt yourself.

Biofeedback

Biofeedback has been found by research and practice to help a person gain a measure of self/body control of many stress-related medical conditions, including chronic pain, headaches, hypertension, Raynaud's phenomenon and anxiety. Biofeedback therapists who have worked with fibromyalgia patients have often helped them to learn how to relax more completely and to decrease their muscle tension. These factors can contribute to a decrease in the patient's level of pain.

When being treated with biofeedback, the patient is hooked up to a sensitive, non-invasive physiological measuring instrument which allows the patient to be made aware of changes in his or her body moment by moment. The therapist then helps the patient to use this unique information to relax and gain additional self/body control.

Biofeedback is one alternative for stress reduction and relaxation and may enhance the effectiveness of your medication.

Tai Chi

Tai Chi is a slow-moving exercise which has been performed for centuries in Asia. Because it is a moving meditation exercise, it gently exercises joints and helps reduce stress. Classes on Tai Chi may be available through local resources such as the Y or Yoga Centers. Instructional videotapes are available in video stores, libraries, or can be ordered through *Yoga Journal.*

Any one of these relaxation techniques could be helpful to those patients who are unable to take medications or for whom the medications provide little relief.

Stress Management Journal

MY STRESSORS	HOW TO AVOID STRESSORS
(Sample) WORK PAIN	*Reduce hours, job training, leave of absence, occupational therapy* *Massage, hot tubs, medicine, exercise, meditation, sleep*

Daily Stress Management Chart

DATE	STRESS (0-10) LEVEL	STRESSORS	SYMPTOMS	COPING METHODS

Personal Activity Chart

TIME	ACTIVITY	SYMPTOMS	STRATEGIES

Managing Unavoidable Stress

▲ Counter stress with activities that reduce your stress level.

Example: Have tea with a friend at a favorite restaurant. Write in your journal everyday. Take a walk on your lunch hour. Close your door and put your feet up for ten minutes. Listen to relaxing, soothing music.

▲ Limit other stresses you have control over.

Example: Postpone dental work. Cancel unnecessary appointments and work tasks. Put off any projects until stress has reduced.

▲ Let go of perfection as a standard for performance for anything that doesn't have to be perfect. We pay an enormous price in terms of time and energy for perfection.

Example: Accept a typewritten letter from your secretary with one typographical error.

▲ Every hour stand up and stretch, do some relaxed breathing, and repeat to yourself a relaxing thought or phrase.

Example: "The day is almost over . . . This project is going well."

▲ Take time for yourself. Sleep in late on Saturday. Relax in a bubble bath at night.

▲ Even though you may have no control over a current stressful event, you can choose how you are going to react to it. You can choose to stay relaxed and take good care of yourself during these difficult periods.

▲ Avoid "catastrophic" thinking such as "this is awful and terrible." This type of thinking only makes matters worse and increases your stress level.

▲ Change negative thoughts into positive ones:

Negative Example: "I'm late and the doctor will be angry for having to wait."

Positive Example: "It's not the end of the world that I'm late. I'll give the doctor's office a call and let them know a problem has come up and they can take the next patient who is waiting."

▲ How important is this anyway? Avoid feeling frustrated over details that in the long run aren't going to matter.

▲ Accept the things you cannot change.

▲ Be flexible and try alternatives which may be less than ideal.

Example: Instead of wrapping up your relative's gift when you are running late, put it into a gift bag or a brown paper bag with a pretty bow!

▲ Delegate tasks whenever possible to family, friends and others. We can't do it all.

▲ Treat yourself gently and with the tender loving care you would treat a friend during stressful times.

▲ Exercise regularly during heavy stress periods to avoid muscle tightness and flare-ups. (Make it a priority.)

▲ Pay attention to sleep habits during high stress times. If sleep quality becomes disturbed, a flare-up might occur. Do all you can to get a good night's sleep (e.g., hot bath and relaxation before bed, shut out noise).

▲ Get extra support. Talk about what is going on, write about it. Look for resources to help you deal with specific problems.

▲ If a stressful situation becomes chronic, get support to make positive changes.

Example: If you have a child who is an alcoholic, try an Alanon support group. Find a marriage counselor to help resolve conflicts in a marriage.

REFERENCES

Alex, Kirsta. *The Book of Stress Survival.* Great Britain: Simon and Schuster, 1986.

Bennett, R. Group treatment of FMS - a 6 month outpatient program, *J Rheumatology*, 23(3):521-8, 1996.

Burns, David D. *Feeling Good: The New Mood Therapy.* New York: Signet, 1980.

Chopra, Deepak. *Quantum Healing.* New York: Bantam, 1990.

Gaston-Johansson F. A comparative study of feelings, attitudes and behaviors of patients with fibromyalgia and rheumatoid arthritis. *Soc Sci Med,* 31, (8):941-947, 1990.

Hart, Archibald. *The Hidden Link Between Adrenalin and Stress.* Dallas Word Publishing, 1986.

Jaffe, Dennis T. *Healing From Within.* New York: Simon and Schuster, 1980.

Kabat-Zinn, Jon. *Full Catastrophe Living.* New York: Dell, 1991.

Nielson, Warren R., Walker, Cathie, McCain, Glenn. Cognitive behavioral treatment of fibromyalgia syndrome: preliminary findings. *Journal Rheum,* 19, 98-103, 1992.

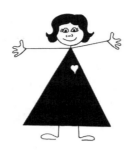

Coping with Psychological Aspects of Fibromyalgia

Recognize Your Feelings

In order to begin to cope with the psychological aspects of this condition, it's important to first accept that "it's not all in your head." Then you can begin to recognize the variety of feelings that you may have over the diagnosis.

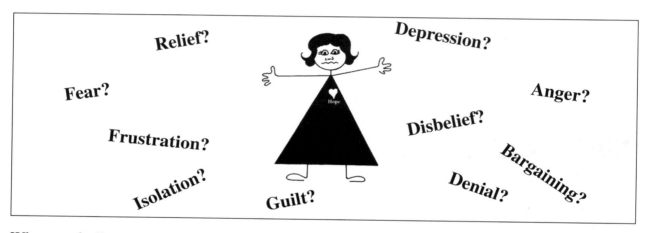

Whatever feelings you might have, it's important not only to recognize them, but to begin to work through them, refocusing your energy on the process of learning to accept or acknowledge your diagnosis. This process takes varying amounts of time for each of us and is often easier said than done. But it's a critical step, because if you stay stuck in the feelings of anger, fear, frustration or denial over your diagnosis, you forego the opportunity of moving on with your life and learning successfully how to cope.

Courage to Change

Your life has changed. You don't have a choice about having fibromyalgia, but you do have choices about how you are going to live with it now that it is a part of your life. One step in beginning to cope might include adopting "The Serenity Prayer":

> *God grant me the serenity to accept the things I cannot change, the courage to change the things I can, and the wisdom to know the difference.*

Reinhold Niebuhr

Since becoming diagnosed with fibromyalgia, you may be faced with changes that you don't want to make, such as pacing your activities, making time for relaxation, aerobic exercise, stretching–the list could go on and on. Instead of resisting change (which is often our first response), try to begin to look at the changes as a positive way of making life easier for yourself, as a way to feel better and as a way to cope more successfully. Sometimes we do need courage to change.

Support

As we make the necessary changes and adjustments, many of us recognize the benefit of having good support. Supportive family members and friends are invaluable and certainly help us to cope. It may be helpful for you to visualize the layers of support that can surround you, as in the diagram on this page. A support journal is also included at the end of this section so that you may write down the specific people, organizations, etc., who form your layers of support.

First Ring

Identify those family members and friends who could provide some support for you. Many people often say that they never would have been able to cope successfully with their fibromyalgia without the support of those closest to them. Do remember, though, to share other parts of your life even when it seems that your world has narrowed to just yourself and your fibromyalgia.

Your health care team can be especially supportive during the initial diagnosis and treatment phase. They are available to answer your questions, to listen, counsel, educate and support you in your quest to cope successfully with the many facets of fibromyalgia.

Second Ring

This second layer of support includes the education you receive in the form of classes, individual instruction, articles, videotapes and books. Counseling and spiritual support can be invaluable in terms of support, and we often encourage individuals to pursue them. Support groups are also beneficial for many people because no matter how much your family and friends love and support you, unless they have fibromyalgia, they really don't know what you're experiencing. Simply the knowledge that you're not alone can make your experience much more bearable. To receive a list of fibromyalgia support groups in your state, contact your local Arthritis Foundation or hospital. The Fibromyalgia Network (602-290-5508) also can provide you with a list of support groups for your state.

Third Ring

Pacing your activities will be helpful in managing fatigue and in creating time to "take care of you." Uplifts are those activities which you enjoy and which give you positive energy. For example, having lunch with a close friend, buying yourself some flowers, going for a walk on a beautiful day, etc. (Further examples of uplifts are found at the end of this section.) By pacing and implementing uplifts, you will create another layer of support for yourself. Being optimistic and having faith in yourself both empower you to seek support, feel supported and extend it to others. These are all part of the process of coping effectively.

Balance

Another method of coping is found in striving to keep one's life in some sense of balance when the pain, fatigue and limitations of fibromyalgia seem to be weighing you down. We can strive to balance the scale by seeking and developing support (as we just discussed), practicing uplifts and taking advantage of those resources that could be helpful. Examples would be massage, a class in water aerobics, a warm water pool, whirlpool, or a new relaxation tape, etc. Develop your own list of resources that work for you, especially when you need to regain some balance. (Refer to list of uplifts at the end of this section.)

Negative   **Positive**

Pain   **Support**
Limitations   **Resources**
Hassles   **Uplifts**

Journaling

Journaling can be a very helpful tool in coping with many of the psychological aspects of fibromyalgia. By writing down your thoughts, feelings, fears, hopes and concerns, you may develop a greater insight, gain a new direction, solve a problem, get in touch with your feelings and/or engage in a rich dialog with yourself. Journaling can also provide an outlet for emotional expression, especially when you ensure that only you will see your thoughts. Repressed or unacknowledged feelings can create a lot of stress and are often expressed in unhealthy, destructive ways. Remember to use the various journal pages included in this handbook to start your own fibromyalgia journal.

Learning to "Take Charge"

A chronic illness like fibromyalgia can foster in patients a sense that they lack control over the status of their health. If they experience little or no control, they can be expected to develop the belief that their health status is controlled by external factors, not by anything the individual might initiate or contribute. From this perspective, the individual with fibromyalgia might feel like a rather passive player in his/her treatment.

It is our belief that you would do well to adopt an active "take charge" role in the management of your fibromyalgia. Your health care team needs to encourage your active participation and respect your questions, comments and suggestions. Your willingness to become educated about fibromyalgia and the various medications and treatments used is the first step in becoming actively involved in your care. It is then your responsibility to participate in the various components of your treatment program and to give feedback and ask questions of your health care team. With this additional input, your treatment program will become more individualized and will likely better fit your needs.

Taking charge of your fibromyalgia is another way of coping with this condition. Remember to be an active participant in your health care, not just a recipient. The choice you make is an important one.

Ask for Help with Problems that You Can't Handle

Unfortunately, no matter how good we are at adjusting to the changes fibromyalgia may bring to our lives, sometimes problems occur that we just can't seem to handle. We may need help in coping and will need to learn when to ask for help. Depression is one of the most common problems in fibromyalgia that one often needs help in managing.

The following are signs of depression:

▲ **Feelings of sadness that last for too long**
▲ **Major changes in sleep habits—sleeping too much or hardly at all**
▲ **Listlessness**
▲ **Poor concentration**
▲ **Major changes in eating habits**
▲ **Sense of worthlessness**
▲ **Severe feelings of guilt**
▲ **Lack of interest in sex**
▲ **Thoughts of or attempts at suicide**

It is important for you to know that depression is a normal part of the grieving process, in this situation, grieving over the loss of health. It is often during this stage that you begin to face the reality of what life is going to be like with fibromyalgia. If you feel unable to gradually arrive at a stage of acceptance and/or feel stuck in a state of depression, it's very important to discuss this issue with a trusted member of your health care team. Depression can lower serotonin and help keep you in a "vicious cycle of pain." It needs to be treated . . . remember to ask for help!

Anxiety and overwhelming stress are also problems that we often can't handle alone. Consulting a psychologist, counselor or psychiatrist can be very beneficial and an important part of your treatment.

In Review, to Cope Effectively:

▲ **Recognize the feelings you have regarding the diagnosis of fibromyalgia.**

▲ **Refocus your energy to the process of learning to accept or acknowledge your diagnosis.**

▲ **Develop courage to change those things that can make your life easier, help you feel better and cope more successfully.**

▲ **Develop a good support system.**

▲ **Strive to keep your life in balance.**

▲ **Use journaling as a way to express your thoughts, feelings, fears, hopes and concerns.**

▲ **Learn to take charge of your fibromyalgia.**

▲ **Ask for help with problems that you can't handle, especially depression.**

Uplifts

Life with chronic pain, fatigue and other symptoms of fibromyalgia can cause one to become discouraged or depressed. **Uplifts** are positive experiences, large or small, which can brighten one's day and make living with pain easier and more bearable. They are personally chosen and meaningful to the person experiencing them.

Make your own list and keep it handy for times when you are in more pain or experiencing discouragement. When the scale is weighing on the negative side, balance the scale by injecting three uplifts into your day to bring the scale to a positive position.

Below are some examples of uplifting possibilities you may wish to do:

▲ take a special coffee or tea break and read a good book

▲ take a walk outdoors on a nice day

▲ call a friend or family member

▲ write in a journal

▲ take a nap

▲ spend time with a favorite friend or support person

▲ go to your favorite floral shop and buy a flower for your desk or table

▲ read a good magazine

▲ take a hot fragrant bath or shower

▲ wear a favorite dress or special soothing perfume

▲ go somewhere you've always wanted to go

▲ learn something new

▲ have a massage or self-massage

▲ write a note to someone expressing how much you care

▲ listen to your favorite music station or tape

▲ do positive self-talks reminding yourself of your specialness and beauty

▲ plan for a goal of something you want to accomplish

▲ plan a vacation or other special occasion

▲ volunteer for a worthy cause

▲ read a book with a child or spouse

▲ ask for a hug from a support person

▲ buy a special treat or present

▲ do some self-care for your pain

▲ go to lunch with a special person

▲ go to a funny or good movie

▲ spend time painting or working on a craft or hobby

▲ do a relaxation exercise with music

▲ swim in a warm pool

▲ have a favorite dinner or other special food

▲ do some simple stretching exercises or other stress-buster exercises

▲ look at a picture book of art, photos, or mementos and reminisce

Support Journal

Write down the specific people, organizations, etc., who form your layers of support. It may give you a better idea of where you could expand your support.

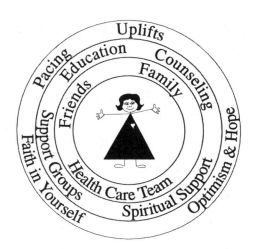

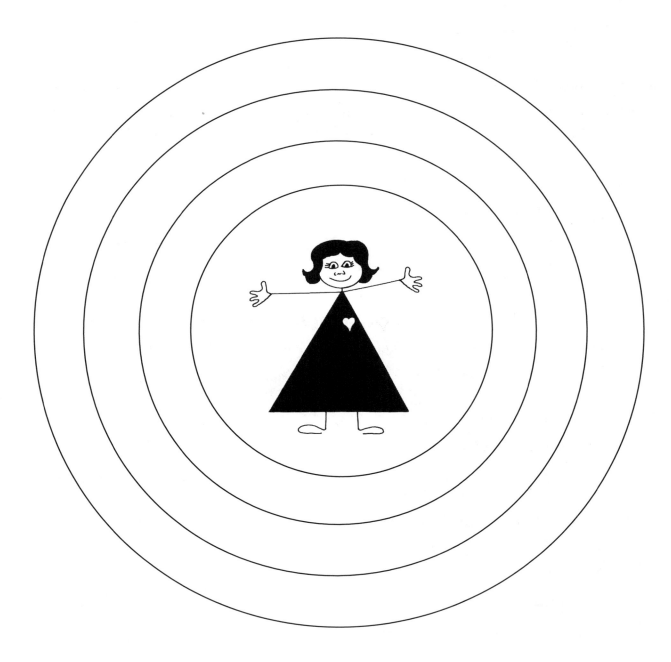

Stress and Coping Resource List

Books

1. *The Big Book of Relaxation* edited by Larry Blumenfeld. Simple Techniques to Control the Stress in Your Life

2. *The Book of Stress Survival* by Alex Kirsta

3. *Coping with Stress, A Guide to Living* by Jane Willard Mills

4. *Feeling Good: The New Mood Therapy* by David D. Burns, M.D.

5. *Fire In the Soul* by Joan Borysenko, Ph.D.

6. *Focus on the Positive - The Workbook* by John Roger and Peter McWilliams

7. *Full Catastrophe Living* by Jon Kabat-Zinn, Ph.D.

8. *Healing from Within* by Dennis T. Jaffe, Ph.D.

9. *Healing Words, The Power of Prayer and the Practice of Medicine* by Larry Dossey, M.D.

10. *I Will Live Today! Affirmations for Strength and Healing While Coping with Serious Illness* by Judith Garrett Garrison, M.Ed., L.S.W., and Scott Sheperd, Ph.D.

11. *Is It Worth Dying For?* by Dr. Robert S. Eliot and Dennis L. Breo

12. *Journey Into Healing* by Deepak Chopra, M.D.

13. *Living with Chronic Illness* by Kathleen Lewis

14. *Living With It Daily - Meditations for People With Chronic Pain* by Patricia D. Neilsen

15. *Meditations for Healing* by Larry Moen

16. *Mind as Healer, Mind as Slayer* by Kenneth R. Pelletier

17. *Minding the Body, Mending the Mind* by Joan Borsyenko

18. *Perfect Health - The Complete Mind/Body Guide* by Deepak Chopra, M.D.

19. *Psychoneuroimmunology: The New Mind/Body Healing Program* by Elliott S. Decher, M.D.

20. *Quantum Healing* by Deepak Chopra, M.D.

21. *Real Magic* by Dr. Wayne W. Dyer

22. *The Relaxation and Stress Reduction Workbook* by Martha Davis, Ph.D., Elizabeth Robbins Eshelmen, M.S.W., and Matthew McKay, Ph.D.

23. *The Relaxation Response* by Herbert Benson

24. *When Bad Things Happen to Good People* by Harold S. Kushner

25. *Why Me, Why This, Why Now?* by Robin Norwood

26. *You Can Heal Your Life* by Louise L. Hay

27. *You Can't Afford the Luxury of a Negative Thought* by Peter McWilliams

Tapes

Music by Stephen Halpern

Various recordings by Whole Person Associates, Duluth, Minnesota

New Age titles

"Renew your Mind and Body" series
These are tapes made specifically for pain and stress reduction.
To order call: (800) 777-8908

"Mindfulness" guided practice tapes with Jon Kabat-Zinn
"Stress Reduction" Series
P.O. Box 547, Lexington, MA 02173
Cost: $11
To order call: (508) 856-0011

"Master Your Mind" by Mary Richards
881 Hawthorne Drive
Walnut Creek, CA 94596
You may request a catalog.
To order call: (800) 345-8515

▲ The tape we often use for demonstration purposes in the class is "Release Discomfort" by Mary Richards. "Relax into Sleep" is another tape by Mary Richards that many enjoy.

Catalogs

Living Arts: (800) 254-8464
This catalog offers a variety of books, CDs, tapes, videotapes and other provisions for yoga, meditations, relaxation, massage, Tai Chi and stress management.

REFERENCES

Backstrom, G., and Rubin, B.R. *When Muscle Pain Won't Go Away.* Dallas, Texas: Taylor Publishing, 1992.

Bishop, G.D., Russell, I.J., Fletcher, E.M., Caro, X., and Wolfe, F. The role of health beliefs in the clinical outcome of fibrositis/fibromyalgia syndrome. (Abstract) University of Texas at San Antonio, 1991.

Gunther, V., et al. Fibromyalgia - the effect of relaxation and hydro galvanic bath therapy on the subjective pain experience. *Clinical Rheumatology,* 13(4):573-8, 1994.

Kaplan, K.H., Goldenberg, D.L., Galvin-Nadeau, M. The impact of a meditation-based stress reduction program in fibromyalgia. *Gen Hosp Psychiatry,* 15(5):284-289, September 1993.

Knipping, Alex, et al. Aspects of coping in fibromyalgia, chronic pain and rheumatoid arthritis. *J Musculoskeletal Pain,* 3(1):102, 1995.

Lewis, K. *Successful Living with Chronic Illness.* Wayne, New Jersey: Avery Publishing, 1985.

Pitzele, S. K. *We are Not Alone: Learning to Live with Chronic Illness.* Minneapolis, Minnesota. Thompson and Company, Inc., 1985.

Register, C. *Living with Chronic Illness: Days of Patience and Passion.* New York: MacMillan, Inc., 1987.

Rotter, J.B. Generalized expectancies for internal versus external control of reinforcement. *Psychological Monographs,* 1960; 80: (1, Whole No. 609), 1960.

White, Kevin P., Nielson, Warren R. Cognitive behavioral treatment of fibromyalgia syndrome: a follow up assessment, *J Rheum,* 22(4):717-721, 1995.

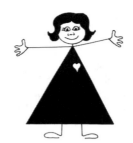

Flare-up Management

The course of fibromyalgia varies from one person to another and is characterized by remissions and flare-ups of symptoms. A remission is defined as a period when one's symptoms are greatly diminished or even absent. Remissions can last for days, weeks, months and even years, often differing from one time to another. A flare-up of symptoms can often be associated with any one or more of the modulating factors that were discussed in the diagnosis and symptoms section (e.g., weather changes, stress, interrupted sleep, depression, postural strain, etc.). Sometimes a flare-up can't be attributed to anything that we're able to identify and can contribute to a feeling of frustration and lack of control over our health. At this point, we need to remember that we can regain a "take charge" attitude over our fibromyalgia and learn to proactively manage the flare-up. The duration, intensity and type of symptoms will often vary and may present us with new challenges. The following management guidelines have been helpful to many experiencing a flare-up and may help you cope more effectively with this distressful part of living with fibromyalgia.

▲ **Remove or change a modulating factor if possible**
  Eliminate or reduce repetitive stress
  Treat other illness
  Correct posture

▲ **Evaluate sleep and discuss other medication options with your physician**
  A different medication or dosage of
  current medication may be increased
  Improve sleep environment

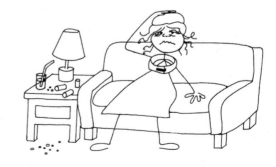

▲ **Relaxation/biofeedback**
  Listen to relaxation tape daily
  Resume practicing of biofeedback

▲ **Rest and be gentle to yourself**
  Take frequent breaks from activity
  Cancel unnecessary appointments
  Give yourself permission to take care of your health
  Try to make activities of daily living as easy as possible
  Take a nap and/or try to get more sleep at night

▲ **Reduce stress level**
  Identify major stressors and eliminate or modify where you can
  (both physical and emotional)
  Alter your perception of the stress when possible
  Journal your thoughts

▲ **Heat/analgesics**

Warm baths/whirlpools/gel packs

Topical capsaicin creams

Short-term use of over-the-counter pain medication can be helpful

▲ **Massage/acupressure/acupuncture**

Use of thera cane and other self-massage tools

Several sessions of physical therapy may be prescribed

See a massage therapist (insurance may cover)

▲ **Gentle stretching**

Often helpful to apply heat for 15-20 min. before stretching

▲ **Decrease duration and intensity of exercise**

Include not only a stretching and aerobic component, but also

a time to sit in a warm bath or whirlpool

▲ **Positive messages**

It's easy to feel discouraged, but try repeating these self-affirming messages:

"I am doing everything necessary to feel better."

"This flare will be over soon."

"I can cope." "I can cope."

▲ **Get extra support during these times from a friend/counselor who understands your illness.**

Flare-ups are a part of living with fibromyalgia. Though they can be frustrating, discouraging and uncomfortable, remember you can help yourself through them by remembering these strategies. You will take charge of fibromyalgia once again!

Journal

(for days that I hurt)

Date: _____

Today I feel: _____

Massage, rest, exercise, heat, cold, relaxation, etc., may help my discomfort today.

    I will do: _____

    When I will do it: _____

Anxiety, a hectic schedule, stress, unresolved conflict, postural strain, etc., may make my symptoms worse. If I am experiencing any of these, I will work on resolving: _____

_____

How? _____

Keeping my mind off of the pain is important. When I'm in pain, I will think about (list some pleasant thoughts and memories): _____

_____

What is something special that I can do for myself today? _____

_____

I need to keep my life focused on healthy habits. A healthy habit that I want to work on is:

_____

I need to keep connected with my family and friends. They are an important support system for me.   I will do: _____

_____

Questions and concerns that I want to remember to ask my doctor or nurse: _____

_____

_____

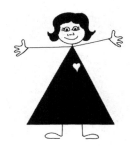

Taking Charge of Fibromyalgia:
A Summary

Because we have given you so much information on how to take charge of your FMS, we realize you are probably feeling quite overwhelmed with your newfound knowledge. To help you feel less overwhelmed, we've broken the steps down so you can quickly see what you need to do in order to **Take Charge of Your Fibromyalgia!**

1. Find a sympathetic and knowledgeable physician.

2. Acknowledge or accept your diagnosis.

3. Educate yourself, your friends, family and co-workers.

4. Begin a fibromyalgia journal.

5. Discuss the need for appropriate medications with your physician.

6. Improve sleep quality.

7. Learn appropriate pain management techniques which you can do yourself at home or at work.

8. Exercise.

9. Eat foods that are high in nutritional value.

10. Learn stress management techniques.

11. Learn to cope with the psychological aspects of living with a chronic illness.

12. Pursue counseling, if necessary.

13. Treat flare-ups quickly.

14. Be assertive in your health care.

15. Use all resources available to you.

16. Pace and balance.

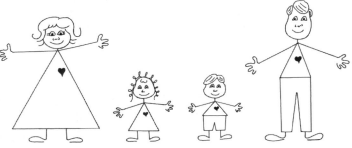

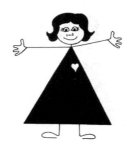

Diet and Nutritional Supplements

- ▲ **Researchers have not focused on this area so far**

- ▲ **Much of this information is taken from anecdotal reports and research prepared by nutritionists, holistic physicians, herbalists, and naturopathic doctors**

- ▲ **We cannot guarantee the benefit of any of these treatments**

- ▲ **A well-balanced diet is important in maintaining a healthy body and mind**

- ▲ **Avoid over-processed foods, nicotine, sugar, caffeine, artificial sweeteners, and preservatives**

- ▲ **Good books are available in health food stores and bookstores**

A number of patients in our classes ask how diet and/or nutritional supplements can help alleviate their FMS symptoms. Although researchers have not focused on this area thus far, some physicians are beginning to assess how vitamin levels, diet changes and food and chemical sensitivities affect certain individuals with FMS. We would like to provide you with an overview of what we have learned about these topics. We would like to emphasize that much of this information has not been subject to rigorous scientific study specifically for FMS. Much is taken from anecdotal reports, nutritionists, herbalists, holistic physicians and naturopathic doctors. We cannot guarantee that any of these nutritional supplements or dietary changes will help your symptoms, although more and more FMS sufferers are turning to this form of treatment when all else fails, or are using it in conjunction with other therapies. We cannot emphasize enough that, for many individuals, treating fibromyalgia requires a multi-treatment approach, and dietary changes could be one piece of the treatment approach that might help you feel better. If there is any possibility that these changes could help you, we do not want to deny you of that information.

Diet

Remember that a well-balanced diet is an important component for good general health. You are what you eat. If you fill your body with poor quality, highly refined, over-processed, foods, nicotine, alcohol, sugar, caffeine, artificial sweeteners, and preservatives, your body will suffer. Some FMS and CFIDS patients have benefited from changing their diets to all fresh, organically produced foods and avoiding the ones just mentioned. There are many good books available that discuss healthy eating. A trip to your local book store will help to educate you in this area.

Food Allergies

▲ **Many FMS patients report sensitivities to foods, drugs, and chemicals**

▲ **Sensitivities can make you feel tired, spacey, flu-like, and have mood changes**

▲ **Laboratory tests are often inconclusive for food allergies**

▲ **Standard elimination diet is effective for detecting food allergies: this diet can be time-consuming and restrictive**

▲ **Try eliminating most common allergy-producing foods**

Many people with FMS feel they have allergies or sensitivities to different foods, drugs and chemicals found in our environment. Some individuals feel so terrible every day, they cannot distinguish which food or chemical could be a potential problem. It might be wise to find a caring physician who can help you determine which, if any, substances you are allergic to. Sensitivities to various substances can make you feel tired, spacey, achy, flu-like, irritable, depressed or can even be life threatening to some sensitive individuals. It may take some time to sort through which substances you are sensitive to, but could be well worth your effort. National sources for physician referrals are listed at the back of this book. Another good place to find a physician in your area is at your local support group.

Standard procedures for detecting food allergies are laboratory tests and the elimination diet method. Because laboratory tests are often not conclusive, some practitioners prefer to use the elimination diet for detecting which food(s) you may be sensitive to. The standard elimination diet consists of lamb, chicken, potatoes, rice, banana, apple and a cabbage family vegetable. Eat only these foods for two weeks. If some of your symptoms disappear, then it might be possible that your symptoms are related to a food sensitivity. If the symptoms do not disappear, it could be that a reaction to one of the foods on the elimination diet is the culprit and you will have to restrict your diet further. Once symptoms have disappeared, specific foods are re-introduced every four days, one at a time. Symptoms will arise if an allergic response occurs. You must be diligent with this method, as it is time consuming and restrictive. An easier approach for the faint-hearted or those not willing to give up so much is to eliminate the most common allergy-producing foods (and usually the ones we like the most), such as milk, wheat, eggs, citrus, sugar, alcohol, chocolate, coffee, and artificial sweeteners such as aspartame (NutraSweet®). It is important to note that if you are allergic to these foods, you may feel worse when you give them up before you feel better (usually a week) as your body goes through a withdrawal period. Some people say they feel a dramatic improvement in the way they feel by detecting and eliminating substances they are allergic to. Before beginning an elimination diet, it is important for you to consult a physician or health professional.

PMS Fibromyalgia Flare and Diet

▲ **Treating PMS or menopausal symptoms might help you feel better**
▲ **Balancing hormones is important**
▲ **Can use prescribed treatments or natural ones**

For those of you whose symptoms flare premenstrually, treating your premenstrual symptoms might help you feel better at this time of the month. Serotonin and estrogen levels are found naturally in reduced levels after ovulation, and some women are especially sensitive to this change in their monthly cycles. Also, women who are premenopausal or experiencing menopause may feel a little better if their hormones can be balanced through proper treatment, either with prescribed hormones or natural treatments. Consult your physician for help in this area. There are many good books on this subject, and they are referenced at the end of this section.

Nutritional Supplements

▲ **Limited research is being done in this area**

▲ **Magnesium, malic acid, and amino acids have been covered in research section**

▲ **FMS and CFIDS newsletters are good sources of information**

▲ **Important to work with a knowledgeable person in this area**

▲ **Resources listed in this book**

Many of our class participants inquire about which nutritional supplements are beneficial for their FMS. There are some anecdotal reports that certain supplements seem to alleviate some people's symptoms. Relief varies from individual to individual, and if supplements help, they often require weeks or months of supplementation. We have already covered magnesium, malic acid, and amino acids in the research section.

FMS and CFIDS newsletters can be good sources for news about nutritional supplementation. Research studies have been few in this area, so much of the available information is experimental. Thomas Romano, M.D., and a few other researchers are finding vitamin deficiencies in some patients and an over abundance of vitamins in others. The B vitamins seem to be the ones found in low levels, while Dr. Romano has found high levels of vitamin A in some of his patients. Other researchers are just beginning to look at vitamin deficiencies; their studies may produce yet another clue to the mysterious puzzle of the FMS syndrome. Dr. Romano has noted that vitamins can be used to correct a nutritional deficiency or imbalance or can be used as pharmacologic agents. Discuss with your physician the need for vitamin levels to be checked and modified. There are blood tests specifically designed to determine vitamin levels which your physician can order for you. Because many physicians are not trained in nutritional therapies, you might have to once again look for someone knowledgeable in this area such as a nutritionist, naturopathic doctor or a holistic physician. Taking vitamins and herbs can be harmful if not used properly and can counteract or interfere with prescribed medications, so it is very important to work with someone who is educated and experienced in this area.

It's important for you to know that water-soluble vitamins, such as the B vitamins, are easily eliminated from the body; therefore it is almost impossible for you to accumulate toxic levels from one or more of these preparations. However, fat-soluble vitamins, such as vitamins A, D, E, and K, can accumulate in the body and exert toxic or untoward effects for many months even after the excess is noted and guarded against. For example, it is known that high levels of Vitamin A in cells can be toxic and can cause muscle pain—a scenario that we need to avoid!

A good book that covers diet, vitamins, herbs and other natural methods is *Chronic Fatigue Syndrome* by Michael T. Murray, N.D., a naturopathic physician who is quite well-known and has published many books on health and healing. Although his book is about CFIDS, many of the remedies could relate to FMS as well. Dr. Jacob Teitelbaum also suggests various vitamins which he uses in his practice for FMS and CFIDS in his book, *From Fatigued to Fantastic!* A good book on herbal therapies is *The Honest Herbal* by Varro Tyler, Ph.D.

David and Margie Squires of Phoenix, Arizona, have started a nutritional supplement company geared specifically for people with FMS and/or Chronic Fatigue Syndrome. They research their supplements and offer high quality vitamins. Information on ordering their catalog and receiving their free newsletter is at the back of this book in the resource section.

Vitamins

Naturopathic physicians and some holistic physicians use nutritional supplements in their practice. To find a qualified physician, contact the American Association of Naturopathic Physicians or the American Holistic Medical Association listed at the end of this section. We have also included a list of supplements reprinted from the newly revised book *Prescription for Nutritional Healing*, by Phyllis Balch, C.N.C., and James Balch, M.D. They have spent years using vitamin and herbal supplements and are widely renowned in the field of nutrition and treating illness with vitamins and dietary changes. You will note that this list is quite long and can be expensive if you choose to try some or all of the suggested supplements.

Although we have included this list for you to refer to, we need to remind you that there are other resources which may suggest even different vitamins for fibromyalgia than this list illustrates. This can be very confusing for FMS patients. Until research is carried out on exactly which specific vitamins are helpful in treating FMS, it is up to you and your physician to use good judgment when making decisions about supplementation.

NUTRIENTS

SUPPLEMENT	SUGGESTED DOSAGE	COMMENTS
Essential		
Coenzyme Q10	75 mg daily.	Improves oxygenation of tissues, enhances the effectiveness of the immune system, and protects the heart.
Acidophilus (Kyo-Dophilus from Wakunaga, Bifido Factor from Natren)	As directed on label.	Candida infection is common in people with fibromyalgia. Acidophilus replaces "friendly" bacteria destroyed by candida. Use a nondairy formula.
Lecithin	As directed on label, with meals.	Promotes energy, enhances immunity, aids in brain function, and improves circulation.
Malic acid and magnesium	As directed on label.	Involved in energy production in many cells of the body, including the muscle cells. Needed for sugar metabolism.
Manganese	5 mg daily. Take separately from calcium.	Influences the metabolic rate by its involvement in the pituitary-hypothalamic-thyroid axis.
Proteolytic enzymes or Infla-Zyme Forte from American Biologics or Wobenzym N from Marlyn Nutraceuticals	As directed on label, 6 times daily, with meals, between meals, and at bedtime.	Reduces inflammation and improves absorption of foods, especially protein, which is needed for tissue repair.
Vitamin A and vitamin E	25,000 IU daily for 1 month, then slowly reduce to 10,000 IU daily. 800 IU daily for 1 month, then slowly reduce to 400 IU daily.	Powerful free radical scavengers that protect the body's cells and enhance immune function. Use emulsion forms for easier assimilation.
or ACES + Zinc from Carlson Labs	As directed on label.	Contains vitamins A, C, and E plus the minerals selenium and zinc, to protect immune function.
Vitamin C with bioflavonoids	5,000–10,000 mg daily.	Has a powerful antiviral effect and increases the body's energy level. Use a buffered form.
Very Important		
Vitamin B complex injections plus extra vitamin B6 (pyridoxine) and vitamin B12 plus raw liver extract	2 cc twice weekly for 1 month or as prescribed by physician. ¼ cc twice weekly for 1 month or as prescribed by physician. 1 cc twice weekly for 1 month or as prescribed by physician. 2 cc twice weekly for 1 month or as prescribed by physician.	Essential for increased energy and normal brain function. Injections (under doctor's supervision) are best. All injectables can be combined in a single syringe.
or vitamin B complex	100 mg 3 times daily, with meals.	If injections are not available, or once the course of injections has been completed, use a sublingual form.
Dimethylglycine (DMG) (Aangamik DMG from FoodScience Labs)	50 mg 3 times daily.	Enhances oxygen utilization by the muscles and destroys free radicals that can damage cells.
Free-form amino acid complex	As directed on label.	To supply protein essential for repair and rebuilding of muscle tissue and for proper brain function. Use a formula containing all the essential amino acids.
Grape seed extract	As directed on label.	A powerful antioxidant that protects the muscles from free radical damage and enhances immunity.
Garlic (Kyolic) plus Kyo-Green from Wakunaga	2 capsules 3 times daily, with meals. As directed on label.	Promotes immune function and increases energy. Also destroys common parasites. To improve digestion and cleanse the bloodstream.
Important		
Calcium and magnesium	2,000 mg daily. 1,000 mg daily.	Needed to balance with magnesium. Needed for proper functioning of all muscles, including the heart; relieves muscle spasms and pain. Deficiency is common in people with this disorder.
or Bone Support from Synergy Plus	As directed on label.	Contains calcium and magnesium plus other minerals to aid absorption.
plus potassium and selenium and zinc	99 mg daily. 200 mcg daily. 50 mg daily. Do not exceed a total of 100 mg daily from all supplements.	Involved in proper muscle function. An important antioxidant. Needed for proper functioning of the immune system.
Capricin from Probiologic	As directed on label.	To combat candida, which is associated with fibromyalgia.
DL-phenylalanine (DLPA)	500 mg daily every other week.	Can be very effective for controlling pain. Also increases mental alertness. Caution: Do not take this supplement if you are pregnant or nursing, or suffer from panic attacks, diabetes, high blood pressure, or PKU.
Essential fatty acids (black currant seed oil, flaxseed oil, and primrose oil are good sources)	As directed on label 3 times daily, with meals.	Protects against cell damage. Helps to reduce pain and fatigue.
Gamma-aminobutyric acid (GABA) or GABA Plus from Twinlab	As directed on label. As directed on label.	For proper control of brain function and to control anxiety. Contains a combination of GABA, inositol and niacinamide.
L-Leucine plus L-isoleucine and L-valine	500 mg each daily, on an empty stomach. Take with water or juice. Do not take with milk. Take with 50 mg vitamin B6 and 100 mg vitamin C for better absorption.	These amino acids are found primarily in muscle tissue. They are available in combination formulas.
L-Tyrosine	500–1,000 mg daily, at bedtime.	Helps to relieve depression and aids in relaxing the muscles. Caution: Do not take this supplement if you are taking an MAO inhibitor drug.
Melatonin	As directed on label, 2 hours or less before bedtime.	Promotes sound sleep. A sustained release formula is best.
Multivitamin and mineral complex plus natural carotenoids (Advanced Carotenoid Complex from Solgar)	As directed on label. 15,000 IU daily.	All nutrients are necessary in balance. Use a high-potency hypoallergenic formula.
Ocu-Care from Nature's Plus	As directed on label.	Contains essential nutrients to protect and nourish the eyes.
Raw thymus and raw spleen glandulars plus multiglandular complex	As directed on label. As directed on label. As directed on label.	To boost the immune system.
Taurine	500 mg daily, on an empty stomach.	An important antioxidant and immune system regulator necessary for white blood cell activation and neurological function.
Vanadyl sulfate	As directed on label.	Protects the muscles and reduces overall body fatigue.

This table is from Prescription for Nutritional Healing, *2nd edition, by James F. Balch, M.D., and Phyllis Balch, C.N.C. Avery Publishing Group, Garden City Park, NY. Reprinted by permission.*

This table is intended for educational purposes only. It is recommended that you discuss all nutritional therapy with your medical advisor. Recommendations will vary from one individual to another.

Herbs

More and more Americans are using natural remedies and flocking to health food stores to buy herbs as well as vitamins. Once again, caution is advised, as some can be toxic, and one can never quite be sure if the actual dosage listed on the bottles is correct. The herbs recommended by *Prescription for Nutritional Healing* for fibromyalgia are:

▲ Astragalus and echinacea enhance immune function.

▲ Black walnut and garlic aid in removing parasites.

▲ Teas brewed from burdock root, dandelion, and red clover promote healing by cleansing the bloodstream and enhancing immune function. Combine or alternate these herbal teas, and drink 4 to 6 cups daily.

▲ Topical applications of cayenne (capsicum) powder mixed with wintergreen oil can help relieve muscle pain. Cayenne contains capsaicin, a substance that appears to inhibit the release of neurotransmitters responsible for communicating pain sensations. Use 1 part cayenne powder to 3 parts wintergreen oil. Cayenne can also be taken orally, in capsule form.

▲ Ginkgo biloba improves circulation and brain function.

▲ Licorice root supports the glandular system.

   Caution: If overused, licorice can elevate blood pressure. Do not use this herb on a daily basis for more than seven days in a row. Avoid it if you have high blood pressure.

▲ Milk thistle protects the liver.

▲ Pau d'arco, taken in tea or tablet form, is good for treating candida infection.

▲ Skullcap and valerian root improve sleep.

This list is from Prescription for Nutritional Healing, *2nd edition, by James F. Balch, M.D., and Phyllis Balch, C.N.C. Avery Publishing Group, Garden City Park, NY. Reprinted by permission.*

▲ St. John's Wort for mild to moderate depression. See your physician.

This is by no means a complete list, although these herbs and vitamin supplements are the ones often mentioned in articles, books and anecdotal reports for treatment of the symptoms of FMS and CFIDS. It is important to note that most of these have not as yet been subjected to scientific studies for fibromyalgia. Some of these herbal preparations take months to work. Be patient. Do your research first so you understand how the herb works.

Adverse Effects of Herbs

The effects of herbs vary according to their potency and the weight, gender, biochemistry, and age of the individual. They also can interact with prescription medications and over-the-counter medications like cough and cold remedies. Herbs are used widely in Europe for medicinal purposes and are fairly safe when taken in appropriate doses. The problem for Americans is that many of our health professionals are not trained in the use of herbs, so we rely on health food store personnel to advise us. Sometimes, these people are not properly trained. So be careful and consult with a knowledgeable practitioner.

Some herbs which are known to be dangerous to take are comfrey, borage, colts foot, crotalaria, senecio, chaparral, germander, jin bu huon (Chinese), ma huang (ephedra), margosa oil, mate tea, mistletoe, pennyroyal, and Tung Shuen.

Hormonal Supplements

▲ **Melatonin helps induce sleep**

▲ **DHEA might improve energy**

▲ **Can purchase over the counter**

▲ **Must be careful as these are potent substances and over-the-counter products are not regulated**

Melatonin

Melatonin is a hormone manufactured from serotonin, secreted by the pineal gland, and is involved in the synchronization of hormonal secretions relating to our sleep-wake cycles. It is stimulated by darkness and suppressed by light. It has been in the news a lot lately, and people are using it as a sleep aid and to help relieve jet-lag. A study in 1973 reported that melatonin supplementation worsened depression in some cases, so if you have trouble with depression, speak to your physician before trying this remedy. It appears that the sleep-enhancing effects of melatonin happen only when melatonin levels are low. It is not like taking a sleeping pill. So, if you have trouble sleeping, do not have depression, and have low melatonin levels, melatonin taken before bedtime might help you fall asleep and stay asleep. The exact dosage to help you sleep is not known, but 3 mg. is more than enough, and some people benefit from dosages as low as .1 mg. Because melatonin is a hormone, it can have very strong effects in the body and should not be used indiscriminately. Just because it is available without a prescription does not mean it is safe, or even that all the uses of it are known. Please be careful when using melatonin and, as always, speak to your physician before using this supplement.

DHEA

Many patients with chronic musculoskeletal problems have low DHEA levels. DHEA (dehydroepiandrosterone sulfate) is an adrenal hormone which has been discussed in the research section. It's been available only by prescription until recently and now can be purchased in many health food stores and some pharmacies. When fibromyalgia patients' DHEA levels were tested, many were found to be low. Supplementing with this hormone has helped some people with FMS feel more energetic. Studies are currently underway to assess DHEA treatment in FMS patients. Consult your physician for the results of these studies.

There is a blood test available to determine your blood level of DHEA, which would help guide your physican in determining what dosage might be best for you. Dr. Thomas Romano states that, "If you have a relatively low DHEA level, then DHEA could be used to bring your blood level into the appropriate range. In this example, the use of DHEA would be the same as using thyroid hormone if someone has a low blood level of thyroid hormone. However, if one wishes to use DHEA if a blood level is not drawn or if the DHEA hormone level is found to be normal, then DHEA is no longer being used as a replacement. In this example, it is being used as a pharmacologic agent to exert specific effects on the human body. Side effects of acne, facial hair growth and oily skin have been reported, but appear to be less common in those patients who have low DHEA levels and are taking this hormone in amounts necessary to replace the body's store of DHEA." Some people report higher levels of energy when taking this supplement, and it is being touted as an anti-aging miracle in magazines and books. Remember, although DHEA is now available without a prescription, it is a potent medication whose long-term effects are unknown. Discuss with your physician what dosage of DHEA would be most appropriate for you; 15-60 mg. is often suggested.

Important Note

▲ **Do not waste your money on "magic cures"**

▲ **Work with a qualified person**

▲ **Discuss all supplements you take with your physician**

Many people have tried various supplements and have spent a lot of money on cures which may or may not benefit you. Please be mindful of this and make wise choices for yourself when using vitamins or herbs, as these can be helpful, yet do have the potential of causing harm. Working with a physician or another qualified person may help alleviate problems that could arise when taking nutritional supplements and/or restricting your diet. Discuss any supplements you decide to take with your physician before taking them. If anyone tells you that they have a particular supplement that will cure you, please beware and do not expect any one supplement to totally resolve your symptoms. If we had found that one supplement, we would all be taking it and be cured! A list of referral resources is listed in the back of this book.

Increasing Serotonin Naturally

Much research has been done on increasing serotonin naturally. There are a few good books available on the subject. These are listed in the resource section at the end of this chapter.

Some methods of increasing serotonin naturally:

▲ **Relaxation, meditation, feeling calm**

▲ **Reducing anxiety**

▲ **Reducing perfectionism and compulsivity**

▲ **Adequate sunlight**

▲ **Adequate exercise: too much depletes serotonin**

▲ **Laughter - having fun!**

REFERENCES

Ali, Majid. *The Canary and Chronic Fatigue.* Life Span Press, 1994.

Balch, James R., Balch, Phyllis. *Prescription for Nutritional Healing.* ($16.95)

Berne, Katrina. *Running on Empty.* Publishers Press, Salt Lake City, 1995. ($14.95)

Brostoff, Jonathan. *The Complete Guide to Food Allergy and Intolerance.* Crown Publishing, 1989. ($15.00)

Courmel, Katie. *A Companion Volume to Dr. Jay A. Goldstein's Betrayal By the Brain.* Haworth Medical Press, 1996.

Dalton, Katherina. *Once A Month.* Hunter House, Inc., 1994. ($11.95)

Dalvitt and McPhillips. The Effect of the Human Menstrual Cycle on Nutrient Intake. *Physiol & Behav.* 31 (2):209-12, Aug. 1983.

DeFeudis. Ginkgo biloba Extract (Egb 761) Pharmacological Activities and Clinical Applications. Elsevier, Paris, France 1991.

Dyons, et al. Serotonin Precursor Influenced by Type of Carbohydrate Meal in Healthy Adults. *American Journal Clin. Nutr.* 47 (3):433-9, March 1988.

Eisinger J. Ayarni, T., Zakarian H, Plantamura A. Thiamin - Dependent Enzymes Abnormalities in Fibromyalgia. *Journal of Musculoskeletal Pain.* Haworth Medical Press, New York, 3:1 p. 112.

Dufty, William. *Sugar Blues.* Warner Publishing, 1975. ($5.99)

Ford, Gillian. *Listening to your Hormones.* Prima Publishing, 1996. (916) 632-4400 ($22.95)

Gerwin R., Gervitz R. Chronic Myofoscial Pain: Iron Insufficiency and Coldness in Risk Factors. *Journal of Musculoskeletal Pain.* Haworth Medical Press, New York, 3:1, p. 120, 1995.

Goldstein, Jay. *Betrayal By the Brain: The Neurological Basisi of Chronic Fatigue Syndrome, Fibromyalgia Syndrome and Related Neural Network Disorders.* Haworth Medical Press, 1996. (800) 342-9678. ($24.95 soft cover) ($39.95 hard cover), plus ($3.00 s&h)

Hugh-Berman, Adriane. *Alternative Medicine: What Works.* Odonian Press, 1996. Box 32375, Tucson, AZ 85751 (520) 296-4056 ($9.00)

Kleijnen J. and Knipschild P. Ginkgo biloba. *Lancet,* 340:1136-9, 1992.

Kotter, I,. Dick, H., and Schweinsberg, F., Soal, J.G. Selenium Levels in Fibromyalgia. *Journal of Musculoskeletal Pain.* Haworth Medical Press, New York, 3:1, p. 46, 1995.

Lark, Susan M. *Chronic Fatigue Self-Help Book.* Celestial Arts, 1995. ($16.95)

Lark, Susan M. *PMS Self Help Book.* P.O. Box 7327, Berkeley, CA, 1993. ($16.95)

Makoul, Sam. Nutrition: Metabolism and Fibromyalgia. *Fibromyalgia Frontiers,* Winter 1996, Vol. 4:1.

Murray, Michael T. *Chronic Fatigue Syndrome.* Prima Publishing, CA, 1994.

Murray, Michael T. *Natural Alternatives to Prozac.* William Morrow & Co., Inc., New York, 1996.

Pfeiffer, Carl C. *Nutrition and Mental Illness.* Healing Arts Press, 1987. ($10.95)

Pierpooli and Regalson. *The Melatonin Miracle.* Simon & Schuster, New York, 1995.

Rector, Linda G. *Healthy Healing, An Alternative Healing Reference.* Page Publications, 1994. ($27.95)

Rogers, S.A. *Tired or Toxic?* Prestige Publishers, 1990.

Romano, T.J. Vitamin A Levels in Patients with Soft Tissue Rheumatism Syndromes. *Journal of Musculosketal Pain,* Haworth Medical Press, New York, 3:1, p. 107.

Russell, I. Jon, Giovengo, S.L. Amino Acids in Cerebrospinal Fluid of Patients with FMS. *Journal of Muskuloskeletal Pain,* Haworth Medical Press, New York, 3:1, p. 9, 1995.

Russell, I. Jon, et. al. Treatment of Fibromyalgia Syndrome with Super Malic: A Randomized, Double-Blinded Placebo Controlled, Crossover Pilot Study, *J. Rheumatology,* 22 (5):953-8, May 1995.

Salmi, H.A. and Sama, S. Effect of silymarin on chemical functional and morphological alterations of the liver. *Scand J Gastroenterol,* 17:517-21, 1982.

Somer, Elizabeth. *The Essential Guide to Vitamins and Minerals.* Harper Collins, 1995. ($17.00)

Somer, Elizabeth. *Food and Mood.* Henry Holt, 1996. ($15.95)

Teitelbaum, Jacob. *From Fatigued to Fantastic!* Deva Press, Annapolis, MD, 1995.

Thorson, Kristin. Does the Food You Eat, Make You Sick? *Fibromyalgia Network,* July 1995.

Tyler, Varro E. *The Honest Herbal & Herbs of Choice.* Pharmaceutical Products Press.

Vliett, Elizabeth. *Screaming to Be Heard: Hormonal Connections Women Suspect and Doctors Ignore.* M. Evans and Company, Inc., New York, 1996.

Waterhouse, Joyce. Novel Treatment Reduces FMS Symptoms. Controlling Food Sensitivities has Wide Impact, *CFIDS Chronicle,* p. 48, Fall 1996.

Weil, A. *Health and Healing.* Houghton Mifflin, Boston, 1988.

Weil, A. *Natural Health, Natural Medicine.* Houghton Mifflin, Boston, 1990

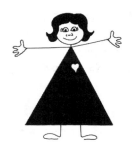

Alternative Treatments: An Overview

Alternative medicine emphasizes wellness and prevention. It uses natural substances to heal and support the body and tries to find causes for health problems in a patient's lifestyle habits, such as diet, stress management, exposure to toxic substances, lack of exercise, and others. Holistic medicine emphasizes a blending of the two, treating the whole person rather than individual symptoms. Alternative medicine is usually less costly than traditional Western medicine, but because many insurance companies do not reimburse for alternative treatments patients must pay out of pocket, which can sometimes prove to be very expensive. Vitamin supplements alone can cost well over $100 per month. Carefully research your alternative treatments and practitioners to make sure you are not wasting your time and money.

Many U.S. physicians claim that much of the research written on alternative medicine is not up to their scientific standards and have, in the past, dismissed the merits of many alternative treatments. Much of the research for these therapies has come from Europe where alternative treatments are more commonly used. At this time, additional research is being carried out in American facilities on some alternative treatments. The government has even opened an Office of Alternative Medicine at the NIH (National Institutes of Health) whose goal is to study alternative medicine. One of the major problems with researching alternative therapies is that natural substances are not patentable, so pharmaceutical companies do not want to waste their time and money on something they cannot patent and benefit from financially.

Some insurance companies are beginning to pay for alternative therapies because they are finding them to be cost-effective. Chiropractic therapy is now covered by 85% of insurance carriers. The FDA recently ruled that acupuncture needles are an approved medical device, so more healthcare plans will be covering that as well. A few plans, mainly on the West Coast, are starting to cover homeopathy, herbs, massage and aromatherapy when referred by a conventional M.D. The state of Washington became the first state to require that health insurance companies cover licensed alternative health care practitioners.

Integrated or holistic health care centers have cropped up in major American cities which offer both allopathic (Western M.D.'s) physicians and alternative therapists, with more scheduled to open up across the country. A few years ago, a Harvard study found that one-third of Americans routinely used alternative therapies, calculating that we spent $14 billion on these therapies in 1990. Physicians were surprised by this report, because most patients do not tell their doctors they are using alternative treatments for fear of criticism or hurting their doctors feelings. In recent years, the American Medical Association passed a resolution encouraging its members to become better informed regarding the technique and practice of alternative care. Many medical schools are now offering classes in alternative therapies, and more research is being carried out in major medical centers, universities and research laboratories.

One of the complaints about alternative therapists is that many are unlicensed. We do need stringent licensing procedures and qualified schools for these therapists because Americans are likely to continue going to see and use these practitioners. Public interest is gaining momentum. You can hardly open up a magazine today and not find many articles on the subject. Licensing would help legitimize alternative therapists.

FMS Patients Seeking Alternative Therapies

We do know that FMS patients are seeking out alternative health-care practitioners. Why? Because we have a chronic condition with no known cure, and many people hope to find a cure somewhere. Oftentimes, patients simply do not like to take drugs and want to use more natural methods to heal their illness. FMS patients' sensitivity to drugs makes us likely candidates for natural substances. We all must remember that many of these alternative therapies have been around for centuries, long before Western medicine. Although a substantial number of FMS patients are trying these therapies, we do not have any hard data on which ones work for which symptoms or how much they help. It is up to you to become better educated in this area. Some patients like the individual attention they receive from alternative practitioners, who are often less harried than M.D.'s who are struggling under time restrictions from managed health-care companies. Many people prefer the holistic approach taken by some M.D.'s who have blended traditional and alternative treatments.

Frustrated with their pain and fatigue and with the slowness of research and development for FMS treatments, some patients are trying remedies which are unproven for FMS. Some people swear that a particular treatment cured them. Because FMS is an individual illness, however, what works for you may not work for others. This variation is true even for the regularly prescribed medications for FMS. Also, be reminded that if a particular supplement truly was the cure for FMS, we would not need to read this book — we would all be cured! Most research shows that FMS sufferers need to change many aspects of their lives and try a variety of treatments in order to feel better. This treatment plan might include dietary changes, exercise, massage, stress management, nutritional supplements, and the use of conventional medicines. Most studies show that one change is not enough to produce benefits.

Be a Wise Consumer

When trying new treatments, be aware that quacks and charlatans do exist. There are desperate people waiting to collect your money, and FMS patients are sometimes desperate! Some will try anything to alleviate their pain. We must be careful and know that some substances are dangerous even though they are natural and sold over the counter. Some alternative treatments lack credentialing organizations and accredited or recognized training institutions. Treatments can range from beneficial to harmless to outright dangerous. They can also be very expensive. Let the buyer beware — educate yourself before you try any remedy.

Conventional drugs, surgeries and treatments can also be dangerous. Some drugs work for some FMS patients, alleviating their pain in varying degrees, improving sleep and lifting mood. Some do not help at all, make us feel worse, or produce intolerable side effects. Just ask any FMS patient who has experienced tricyclic hangover, heart palpitations, increased pain, weight gain, ulcers, insomnia or depression from one of the commonly prescribed medications for FMS. How many people have had needless surgery for back pain that continued to exist after the surgery? Conventional medicine is not 100% either.

If the American public continues to use alternative therapies, more will be available, more and better research will be conducted, and allopathic and alternative therapists will discontinue their cold war and work together in improving our health.

For information from The Office of Alternative Medicine, write:
National Institutes of Health
Alternative Medicine
P.O. Box 8218
Silver Springs, MD 20907-8218
Tel: (301) 402-2466
Toll-free: (888) 644-6226

Glossary of Alternative Therapies

Following is a brief description of the better known alternative therapies and national numbers to call for information on each one.

Acupressure – Manual application of pressure with fingertips at points where acupuncture needles would be inserted, according to the same principles by which acupuncture operates. American Oriental Bodywork Therapy Association, Glendale Executive Campus, Ste. 510, 1000 White Horse Road, Voorhes, NJ 08043; (609) 782-1616.

Acupuncture – Ancient Chinese medical treatment based on the belief that the body has a number of meridians that conduct energy throughout the body. Symptoms result from a blockage in these meridians. The treatment consists of inserting fine needles, sometimes along with heat, electricity, herbs, oils or lasers, at various points along the body's meridians chosen to alleviate blockages for specific symptoms. Its mechanism of action is not completely understood but is believed to stimulate endorphins (pain killers) and serotonin. The FDA has recently approved acupuncture needles as safe medical devices. American Academy of Medical Acupuncture, 5820 Wilshire Blvd., Ste. 500, Los Angeles, CA 90036; (213) 937-5514, (800) 521-2262.

Applied Kinesiology – A system of testing muscle strength developed by chiropractors. An applied kinesiologist uses procedures that strengthen weak muscles and relax tense muscles. This helps rebalance an out-of-balance body. Allergies and vitamin deficiencies are also detected and treated using this method. International College of Applied Kinesiology, P.O. Box 905, Lawrence, KS 66044; (903) 542-1801

Aromatherapy – A holistic therapy that uses essential oils derived from plants to restore the body's health through the sense of smell. These oils are either inhaled, put in bath water, massaged into the skin or diffused into the air. National Association for Holistic Aromatherapy, P.O. Box 17622, Boulder, CO 80308; (800) 566-6735.

Ayurveda – Ancient system of Indian holistic medicine based on the Hindu scriptures. It is based on the three doshas called vata, pitta and kapha. Each person has a predominant dosha or combination. Imbalances in these can cause ill health. The Ayurvedic practitioner uses foods, herbs, meditation and exercise to correct imbalances. Maharishi Ayur-Veda Association of America, P.O. Box 282, Fairfield, IA 52556; (515) 472-8477.

Chiropractic – Illness is believed to stem from misaligned joints or vertebrae, preventing transmission of signals between the brain and the rest of the body. Chiropractic physicians manually manipulate the spine and joints to improve alignment. It is the second most prevalent form of therapy after conventional medicine. Many chiropractors offer nutritional counseling as well as kinesiology, craniosacral work and massage therapies as adjuncts to manual manipulation. American Chiropractic Association, 1701 Clarendon Blvd., Arlington, VA 22209; (703) 276-8800, (800) 986-4636.

Hands-on Healing – Essentially, any treatment using a laying on of hands (although there does not actually have to be touching) by healers who act as channels to harness spiritual, God-given universal healing energy. The American Holistic Nurses Association has done studies in this area and has found evidence that some form of change does take place in the patients' body (via studies done in blood) when this technique is employed. There are many branches of this therapy: Reiki, Therapeutic Touch, Omega Healing, followers of Barbara Brennan (a healer and former NASA physicist), Renewal therapy, Polarity, Mari-El, Shiatsu and others. Touch for Health Association, 6955 Fernhill Drive, Malibu, CA; (800) 466-TFHA; Reiki Alliance, P.O. Box 41, Cataldo, ID 83810; (208) 682-3535.

Holistic Medicine – Any system of medicine that considers the whole person: physically, mentally and emotionally. It treats not only the diseased area, but strives to heal underlying causes. American Holistic Medical Association, 4101 Lake Boone Trail, Ste. 201, Raleigh, NC 27607; (919) 787-5181.

Homeopathy – Samuel Hahnemann developed homeopathic medicine over 200 years ago in Germany. He coined the phrase "Let like be treated by likes," or the Law of Similars. It is based on the assumption that a substance that provokes symptoms in a healthy person cures those same symptoms in a sick person, and the more diluted the dose, the greater its efficiency in helping the body heal itself. The remedies, as they are called, are inexpensive and can often be found in local health food stores. There are homeopathic physicians in some areas of the U.S., although many more are found in Europe. National Center for Homeopathy, 801 N. Fairfax Street, Ste. 306, Alexandria, VA 22314; (703) 548-7790.

Magnetic Therapy – The use of magnets to improve energy and blood flow in the body. Our bodies are surrounded by magnetic fields which affect us according to weather changes, the earth's magnetic fields, power lines and electrical appliances. There are magnetic strips, pillows, mattresses, and shoe inserts. These are placed on the body in areas where there is pain and are supposed to improve blood flow to that area. Some physicians are beginning to use them in their practices. You can purchase them through catalogs or one of the multilevel marketing organizations. For a catalog call or write: Mid-American Marketing Corp., P.O. Box 124, Eaton, OH 45320; 800-922-1744.

Naturopathy – Uses the body's self-healing system to repair itself. Only natural therapies are employed: fasting, organic foods, water therapy, aromatherapy, massage, osteopathy and supplements. American Association of Naturopathic Physicians, 2366 Eastlake Avenue East, Ste. 322, Seattle, WA 98102.

Reflexology – Restoring health through the massaging of specific areas in the feet and hands. Certain points on the feet are thought to correspond to organs and other areas of the body. International Institute of Reflexology, P.O. Box 12642, St. Petersburg, FL 33733-2642 ; (813) 343-4811.

ALTERNATIVE

REFERENCES

Hugh-Berman, Adriane. *Alternative Medicine: What Works.* Odonian Press Tucson, AZ, 1996 $12.75 (800) 788-3123.

Murray, Michael T. *Chronic Fatigue Syndrome.* Prima Publishing, California, 1994.

Murray, Michael T. *Natural Alternatives to Prozac.* William Morrow & Company, Inc. New York, 1996.

Natural Health, April 1996. Boston Common Press. Brookline Village, MA.

Pellegrino, Mark. *The Fibromyalgia Survivor.* Anadem Publishing, Columbus, OH, 1995.

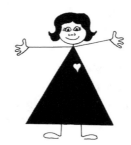

Pioneering Treatments

▲ **Some physicians have been using treatments not yet thoroughly researched**

▲ **Trying one of these treatments should be done with extreme caution**

▲ **These physicians use a variety of tests, medications, vitamins, and hormones**

▲ **Many of their patients do well**

▲ **Read about their treatments in our book, their books, in FMS newsletters or the *CFIDS Chronicle***

▲ **Share this information with your physician**

▲ **Contact them personally**

There are some physicians who have been treating FMS patients by using therapies which could be described as "experimental." These treatments have not been subjected to scientific study at this time (although some are in the process of being researched and others will be studied in the future). We would like to share with you a few of the more widely recognized physicians performing this type of pioneering work, because we feel that this information should be freely accessible to all FMS sufferers. If you choose to try some of these therapies, you might have to find a physician in your area willing to accommodate you. Remember that trying a novel therapy should be done with extreme caution. The authors are not claiming to provide all the necessary information needed to provide these treatments in this book, but are giving an overview of the main points of these treatments. The physician protocols are listed in the appendix at the back of the book. For those interested in using their treatments, purchasing the physician's book or contacting them personally is needed to acquire the correct protocol.

Dr. Jacob Teitelbaum is one such physician. He suffers from CFIDS and FMS and knows firsthand how it affects someone. We have already made reference to his book which describes in accurate detail his treatment protocol for FMS and CFIDS. Dr. Teitelbaum has provided a synopsis of his protocol in the appendix. He uses various laboratory diagnostic tests to assess a number of problems he feels contribute to FMS and CFIDS. After he takes a complete history, he may treat you with some or all of the following: synthroid or armour thyroid to boost a low thyroid level, cortef for an adrenal insufficiency, DHEA to boost DHEA levels, medications to treat neurally mediated hypotension which causes dizziness, oxytocin (a female hormone), estrogen and progesterone, various vitamins, anti-depressants, herbals for sleep aids, anti-yeast treatments, stool parasite therapies, homeopathics and various other medications such as nitroglycerin, naphazoline hydrochloride (eye-drops), calcium channel blockers, and others.

Dr. Teitelbaum's treatment program has benefited many patients and takes into account the fact that FMS symptoms may be caused by a combination of factors. He is in the process of researching his treatment protocol; results should be available in 1998. You may want to purchase his book and share it with your own physician who might be interested in trying these treatments. He also offers a newsletter. Ordering information is listed in the resource section.

Dr. Jay Goldstein is another physician and researcher whom we have mentioned previously in the research section. He has been treating FMS and CFIDS patients for over 15 years and has written a book geared for the physician called *Betrayal By the Brain: The Neurologic Basis of Chronic Fatigue Syndrome, Fibromyalgia Syndrome and Related Neural Network Disorders.* He also offers a companion book written by a patient for patients which you can also order, called *A Companion Volume to Dr. Jay A. Goldstein's Betrayal By the Brain,* by Katie Courmel. Information on ordering is located in the resource section. His treatment protocol differs substantially from those who use medications to alleviate only specific symptoms, such as low serotonin levels. He believes FMS and CFIDS patients suffer from problems in the way their brains process sensory input from noise, lights, odors, pain, food, medications, and chemicals. By a complex mechanism involving various brain chemicals, our brain interprets information it receives from our environment, filters out appropriate and inappropriate information, and tells our body how to handle the input. Dr. Goldstein feels our brains are misinterpreting the information, resulting in an amplification of pain signals, odors, and other sensations. Just going to the local mall bombards our senses with so much stimuli it can prove exhausting. This "wears" out the brain and can cause the cognitive problems many experience.

Goldstein believes FMS and CFIDS patients have a genetic predisposition for developing these syndromes. Developmental issues, in which one feels unsafe for a period of time causing a hypervigilant attitude, can change the way the brain responds to stimulus; exposure to viruses, severe emotional stress and exposure to environmental stressors, are all factors in the development of these syndromes. Some people may be particularly strong in their genetic predisposition and will develop these syndromes no matter what their stressors may be, while others need a variety of these stressors to occur before they will develop FMS or CFIDS. Dr. Goldstein treats his patients in a very different manner than other physicians. A synopsis of his treatment protocol is listed in the appendix at the end of the book. You will note that he uses a variety of medications. Once again, your own physician might be interested in trying this treatment protocol, or you can contact Dr. Goldstein personally.

Specific Treatments

- ▲ Oxytocin • DHEA • Nitroglycerin
- ▲ Atenolol • Florinef • Increase salt and water
- ▲ Guaifenesin
- ▲ Intravenous ketamine
- ▲ Anti-yeast treatments
- ▲ Decompression surgery of craniovertebral stenosis
- ▲ Biofeedback and EEG treatment
- ▲ Balancing dopamine and serotonin

Oxytocin • DHEA • Nitroglycerin

Another therapy that has proven beneficial to some patients in conjunction with other treatments described is that used by Jorge Flechas, M.D., Jay Goldstein, M.D. and Jacob Teitelbaum, M.D. We have already mentioned that DHEA levels were found to be low in FMS patients. By carefully listening to his patients' complaints, Dr. Flechas decided that the hormone oxytocin, along with DHEA supplementation, might help alleviate some of his patients' symptoms. He first runs a blood test to determine baseline DHEA levels, then adds supplements to bring levels up to what they should be at around age 30 (150-200 mcg./dl.); 25-50 mg. of DHEA is recommended, either in capsule form or cream. Dosages need to be determined by a physician as DHEA does have side effects, and long-term usage has not yet been determined. Checking estrogen and testosterone levels is also recommended.

Once your DHEA is up to optimal levels, Dr. Flechas tries his patients on a 10 ml. injection of oxytocin. Oftentimes patients will notice a flushed feeling in their hands or face immediately after the injection, which may or may not last for more than a few minutes. Positive effects will take approximately two weeks. Dr. Flechas recommends taking supplements of choline and inositol to increase the effectiveness of the oxytocin. Nitroglycerin is another medication he adds to his regime to enhance pain relief. Patients who benefit from this treatment often have cold hands and feet and are pale. Daily injections of oxytocin can be given, or there is a capsule available from the pharmacies listed in the appendix. Dr. Goldstein believes injections are more effective. (One can learn to give oneself injections.)

Not much has been written about oxytocin in the literature, but it is known to have a role in inducing labor in pregnant women, facilitating the let-down response in lactating women, and regulating blood circulation in the small vessels of the body. It also has an analgesic effect, raises sex-drive levels, affects concentration, is released during orgasm, and performs a host of other functions. This hormone works within a complex network of other chemicals in our bodies that have been found to be dysregulated, such as neuropeptide Y, corticotropin releasing hormone (CRH), thyroid hormone, estrogen, DHEA, and others.

Two of the side effects are weight gain and water retention. No studies have been performed on this hormone treatment as of yet, but will hopefully be forthcoming.

PIONEERING

Atenolol • Florinef • Increase Salt and Water Intake for Neurally Mediated Hypotension

If you are troubled by dizziness, and/or fainting spells you might want to speak to your physician about the possibility of having a cardiologist perform a tilt-table test. During the test you are strapped to a table and turned 70 degrees so that your legs are close to the floor but do not touch it. Normally, when you get up from a sitting position your brain signals your blood pressure to perform properly when your feet touch the ground. Researchers have found that CFIDS patients and some FMS patients have a dysfunction in the regulation of this system and their blood pressure drops significantly, causing improper blood flow to the brain. This dysfunction can lead to feelings of fatigue and other symptoms associated with FMS/CFIDS. These tests were originally performed by Johns Hopkins University researchers and replicated by Daniel Clauw, M.D., of Georgetown University. A natural treatment for this problem consists of increasing salt intake and drinking lots of water. Some physicians prescribe atenolol (Tenormin), a beta-blocker, or Florinef (fludrocortisone), an adrenal steroid. These drugs do have side effects which your physician should make you aware of.

You could have this condition even if you do not have low blood pressure or a history of fainting or dizziness. This treatment is well worth pursuing and might be a good addition to your overall program.

Guaifenesin

Dr. St. Armand of Marina Del Ray, California, has been using guaifenesin, an ingredient found in the cough medicine Robitussin. Theorizing that FMS patients have a genetically inherited defect in how their bodies excrete phosphates, Dr. St. Armand found that pure guaifenesin works on the kidneys to increase removal of phosphates through the urine. He has treated over 3,000 patients in this manner and claims to have had good results. But, when Dr. Robert Bennett performed a year-long placebo-controlled trial of guaifenesin, guaifenesin proved to be ineffective. In his study, twenty FMS patients were given 600 mg. of guaifenesin twice a day and another twenty patients were given a placebo twice daily. None of the forty patients knew if they were taking guaifenesin or the placebo. All were instructed not to take salicylates because they interfere with the functioning of guaifenesin. Dr. Bennett found that none of his study variables changed significantly over the year and that the response to guaifenesin was the same as that for the placebo. Obviously, Dr. St. Armand and Dr. Bennett disagree on the usefulness of this compound. Dr. St. Armand believes Dr. Bennett's results were not positive because salicylates, a common ingredient in cosmetics, aspirin and herbal medications, were not totally excluded from the study and rendered the guaifenesin treatment ineffective.

The guaifenesin controversy has intrigued many and may be further studied in the future. At this time, its effectiveness is certainly questioned.

Intravenous Ketamine

One study using intravenous morphine, lidocaine and ketamine showed that ketamine proved to be the most effective in reducing pain levels. Morphine, an opiod, did not help at all in this study; lidocaine, an anaesthetic used in trigger point injections, was somewhat helpful; and ketamine, an NMDA pain receptor antagonist, decreased pain and had a longer lasting effect than the others. With its promising results, this study could help lead researchers to other drugs which affect the NMDA receptors and possibly help alleviate pain for FMS patients.

Anti-Yeast Treatments

Some physicians and holistic practitioners believe there is an underlying yeast problem contributing to FMS/CFIDS symptoms. The most common yeast, *candida albicans*, is thought to be the culprit. Finding a physician to treat yeast problems can be difficult, however. Many holistic doctors treat for candida, as do many nutritionists and Chinese medicine doctors. Nutritionists cannot prescribe anti-fungal medications but will use various herbs, vitamin supplements and changes in diet to help alleviate yeast overgrowth. Some physicians, such as Jacob Teitelbaum, M.D., whose book is referred to in our resource list, use both to rid patients of yeast overgrowth.

Our bodies naturally have yeast living in harmony with friendly bacteria inside our bodies. Yeast are there to help our bodies in various ways, but sometimes the yeast overpower the "good bacteria" and cause a yeast invasion. This can occur after repeated courses of antibiotics. Yeast also thrive on sugar and yeast-laden foods such as cheese, bread, and wine. Giving up sugar and all sugar-containing products, including corn syrup, jelly and honey, is the recommended treatment for controlling a candida overgrowth. Some practitioners recommend giving up all yeast-containing foods such as cheese, beer, wine, and bread. Others feel that giving up sugar only is sufficient. Your body will most likely go through a withdrawal period in the first seven to ten days of a diet like this; you may even feel worse as the yeast die off because their source of "food" has been removed. Many people are amazed how their craving for sugar decreases if they can abstain from sugar for just ten days. Believe it or not, you may not even want sugar anymore! It is also recommended to replace the friendly bacteria that have been lost, by taking acidophilus supplements or eating plain yogurt (without sugar) which contains live acidophilus cultures.

It is very important to read labels on all foods you buy if you choose to eliminate sugar. Many foods we buy today include sugar disguised as high fructose corn syrup, dextrose, and maltose. Many cereals are loaded with sugar, as are some breads. Shopping in a health food store or buying bread from a bread maker who uses only stone ground grains and adds no sugar is advised. Some grocery store chains are offering more sugar-free selections as consumers are becoming more health conscious. Remember, just because a label says "all natural" or "no artificial ingredients" does not mean the product hasn't been sweetened with fruit juices, which you may need to avoid, too. Because fruits and fruit juices contain naturally occurring sugars, some health practitioners recommend giving these up for a time, as well. You may need six to twelve months on this diet to take care of the yeast overgrowth. That may sound like a long time, but it can be well worth the trouble if you feel better in the future.

Laboratory tests for detecting yeast overgrowth are not thought to be conclusive, so many practitioners use symptoms and questionnaires to determine whether or not the problems you are having are yeast related. Your physician can prescribe the anti-fungal medications for you, and you could refer to Dr. Teitelbaum's book for his protocol in using this type of therapy. The medications commonly used to treat fungal overgrowth are Diflucan, Sporanex, and Nystatin. There are new ones coming on the market in the future. William Crook, M.D., has written two books on yeast problems and treatments which are listed in the references at the end of this section.

Decompression Surgery of Craniovertebral Stenosis

Michael J. Rosner, M.D., a neurosurgeon at the University of Alabama in Birmingham, has found that some patients with FMS or CFIDS suffer from some element of craniovertebral compression. Symptoms associated with this are similar to FMS/CFIDS symptoms and may include: headaches, neck pain, upper and lower extremity pain, burning, a feeling of tightness, numbness, clumsy hands, stiffness, spasticity, atrophy, flushing, sweating, uninary frequency, irritable bowel, burning feet, dizziness, sore throats, blurred vision and cognitive problems. Spinal cord compression can occur from a congenital cervical stenosis, from an accident where the neck is hyperextended, after surgery, or after a viral infection. Abnormal findings in a neurological exam may indicate this condition; an MRI is needed to confirm it. Dr. Rosner states that numbness, weakness and imbalance are particularly important symptoms to note in evaluating this condition.

Dr. Rosner has found that a number of patients with FMS or CFIDS who suffer from craniovertebral compression respond favorably to decompression surgery of craniovertebral stenosis. This procedure involves a laminectomy and relieves the pressure from the spinal cord, improving the flow of spinal fluid. Over 50% of his patients reported that many of their symptoms improved from this surgery. Symptom improvement after surgery was:

headache	88%	memory	62%
sore throat	72%	bowel	57%
joint pain	82%	bladder	70%
muscle pain	80%	balance	78%
grip	75%		

Conservative treatment for this condition consists of limiting neck hyperextension and flexion by wearing a cervical collar. Supporting your neck during the night with proper cervical pillows may also be helpful, along with physical therapy and improving one's posture.

This is yet another potential problem that may be contributing to some patients' symptoms. You may want to discuss this possibility with your physician.

Biofeedback and EEG Treatment

Stuart Donaldson, Ph.D., of Calgary, Alberta, Canada, has been treating patients with a combination of biofeedback and EEG brain wave therapy which uses no drugs and has shown to be helpful in reducing symptoms.

Balancing Dopamine and Serotonin

Dr. Daniel G. Malone, M.D., a rheumatologist at the University of Wisconsin, has been treating FMS patients with a combination of dopaminergic and serotonergic drugs including: L-dopa, 5-hydroxy tryptophan (5 HTP), Fenfluramine, Pemoline and phentermine. He found statistical improvement in 76 patients out of 122 using this protocol. Unfortunately, two of the medications he had been using, fenfluramine and phentermine, have been withdrawn from the market because of serious heart-valve complications found in some patients who were taking these medications for weight loss.

Important Note

We believe these novel treatments are exciting to report on because they add to the possibilities of treatments for improving your symptoms. Some of your physicians may not know about these therapies, so it might be up to you to educate your physician. Dispensing this information to all physicians involved with FMS and CFIDS patients is important in providing helpful treatment. Because these treatments are so new, it is not known whether they are beneficial when prescribed singly or in conjunction with other treatments. These treatments have not been subjected to research as of yet, and using them may be risky for you. It might be something you could look into, however, if the other, more researched treatments described in this book have been tried and you still do not feel better. Many physicians feel a multi-disciplinary treatment approach is necessary to control FMS, which means using all, many, or some of the treatment options described in this book. At this time, we still do not have a "magic" pill which cures all the symptoms of FMS, but at least we have more treatment options to choose from than we did two or three years ago. We, the authors, feel we have covered the major new treatments available at this time, although we do not claim to have knowledge of all treatments which are being carried out at this point in time. Please call or write to us if you know of any treatments you feel are worth reporting.

REFERENCES

Bon-Holaigah, et al. The Relationship Between Neurally Mediated Hypotension and the Chronic Fatigue Syndrome. *JAMA*. 274:961-967, 1995.

Bruno, Richard L. Fainting and Fatigue, Causation or Coincidence? *The CFIDS Chronicle*. pp. 37-39, Spring 1996.

Carpman, Vicki L. Cough Syrup for Pain? Does Unique Treatment Reverse FMS/CFIDS? *The CFIDS Chronicle.*, pp. 46-47, Fall 1996.

Chafety. *Nutrition and Neurotransmitters: The Nutrient Basis of Behavior.* Englewood Cliffs, NJ, 1990.

Crook, William. *The Yeast Connection and the Woman.* Professional Books, Inc., 1995.

Crook, William. *CFIDS and the Yeast Connection.* Professional Books, Inc., 1992.

Epstein, J.A., Carros, R., Hyman, R.A., Costa, S. Cervical myelopathy caused by developmental stenosis of the spinal cord. *J. Neurosurg,* 51:362-369, 1979.

Gerwin R. A Study of 96 Subjects Examined Both for FMS and Myofascial Pain. *Journal of Musculoskeletal Pain.* Haworth Medical Press, New York, 3:1, p. 121, 1995.

Goldstein, Jay. *Betrayal By the Brain: The Neurological Basis of Chronic Fatigue Syndrome, FM Syndrome and the Related Neural Network Disorders.* Haworth Medical Press, New York, 1996.

Karoliussen, O.H., Kvlheim, L. Effects of Mexiletine on Pain and other Symptoms in Primary Fibromyalgia. *Journal of Musculoskeletal Pain,* 3(1), 26, 1995.

Langfitt, T.W. Cervical spondylosis: the neurological mimic. *W.V. Med J,* 65:97-100, 1969.

Malone, Daniel G. Treatment (RX) of 76 patients with primary fibromyalgia (1^O FM) with combined dopaminergic and serotonergic drugs. Poster, ACR Annual Convention, 1996, Orlando, Florida.

Meholic, T.F., Pezzuli, R.T., Applebaum, B.I. Magnetic resonance imaging and cervical spondylotic myelopathy. *Neurosurgery,* 26:217-227, 1990.

Murone, I. The importance of the sagittal diameters of the cervical spinal canal in relation to spondyloses and myelopathy. *J Bone Joint Surg,* 56 B:30-36, 1974.

Rosner, M.J., Banner, S.R., Guin, S., Oper, A.R., Johnson, A.H., Rosner, A.D., Wadlington, V. Response of the cervical spinal cord to decompression for congenital cervical stenosis. Submitted to *Neurosurgery,* 1997. Reference I.D. #2838.

Rowe, P., et al. Is Neurally Mediated Hypotension an Unrecognizable Cause of Chronic Fatigue? *Lancet,* 345:623-24, March 11, 1995.

Rowe, Peter C., Calkins, Hugh. NMH: One Year Later. Johns Hopkins Research Update. *The CFIDS Chronicle,* pp. 49-50, Fall 1996.

Russell, I. Jon, Gilbert,V., Goldstein, Jay. Could low levels of cerebrospinal fluid endothelin explain the vasoconstrictive response seen in pre- and post-treatment brain spect of CFIDS/FMS patients? *Journal of Musculoskeletal Pain,* 3(1), 14, 1995.

Sinclair, David J., et al. Interdisciplinary Treatment for Fibromyalgia: Treatment Outcome and 6 Month Follow-up. 388. Scientific Abstracts. ACR Annual Meeting. October 1996.

Sletvold, M., et al. Information Processing in Primary Fibromyalgia, Major Depression and Healthy Control, *J. Rheumatology* 22 (1):137-42, January 1995.

Teitelbaum, Jacob. *From Fatigued to Fantastic!* Deva Press, Annapolis, MD, 1995.

Thorson, Kristin. *Fibromyalgia Network*, October 1995.

Thorson, Kristin. *Fibromyalgia Network*, January 1996.

Thorson, Kristin. *Fibromyalgia Network*, April 1996.

Thorson, Kristin. *Fibromyalgia Network*, January 1997.

Welin, M., Lownertz, M.L., Bragee, B. Is the pain in Fibromyalgia NMDA-receptor Mediated? *Journal of Musculoskeletal Pain,* 3(1), 8, 1995.

PIONEERING

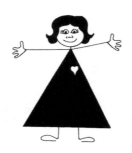

Treatment Pyramid

Comprehensive Treatment for Fibromyalgia Syndrome

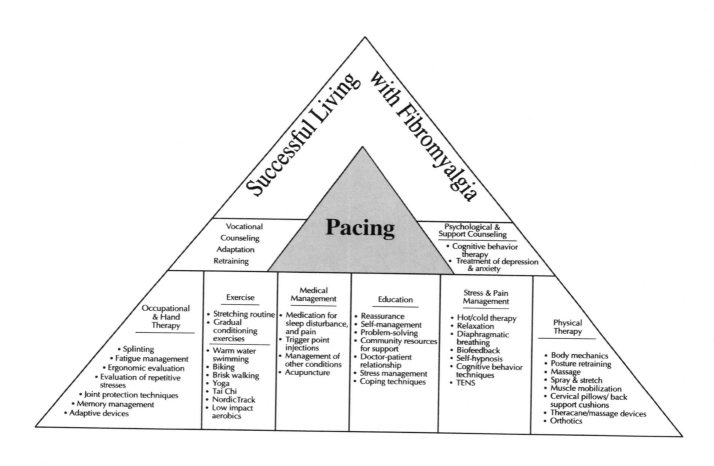

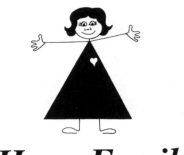

Hope Family

Healing begins with hope.

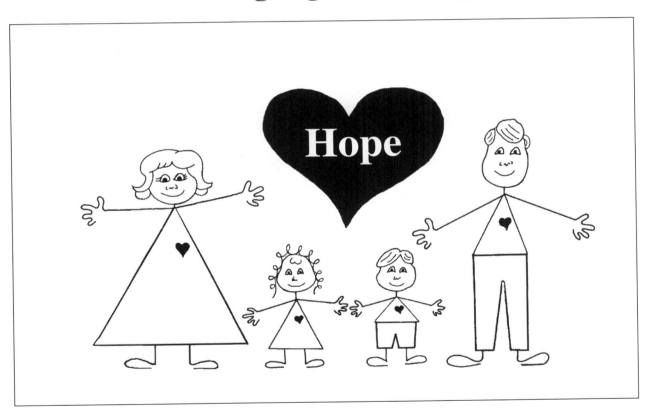

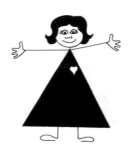

Resources

Books and Publications

Betrayal by the Brain: The Neurological Basis of Chronic Fatigue Syndrome, Fibromyalgia Syndrome and Related Neural Network Disorders by Jay A. Goldstein, M.D. This book discusses the latest research and discoveries by Dr. Goldstein on neurosomatic disorders. It is recommended reading for health professionals and neuroscientists, $29.95 + $4.00 shipping and handling. Haworth Medical Press, 10 Alice Street, Binghamton, NY 13904; (800) 342-9678, fax (800) 895-0585.

Chronic Fatigue Syndrome: Charting Your Course to Recovery by Mary O'Brien, M.D. 93-page book by a physician who shares her personal story of living with CFIDS and overcoming its debilitating effects. Specific treatment options and self-help steps are also discussed, $14.25 + $3.50 shipping and handling. Anadem Publishing Inc., 3620 North High Street, Columbus, OH 43214; (800) 633-0055, fax (614) 262-6630.

Chronic Illness and Uncertainty by Don. L. Goldenberg, M.D. This new book discusses the diagnosis and management of fibromyalgia, chronic fatigue, migraine, insomnia, chronic back pain and depression, $16.50 + $3.50 shipping and handling. Dorset Press, P.O. Box 620026, Newton Lower Falls, MA 02162, (617) 969-5286.

The Chronic Pain Control Workbook: A Step-by-Step Guide for Coping With and Overcoming Pain by Ellen Mohr Catalano, M.A., and Kimeron N. Hardin, Ph.D. The authors collaborated with an eight-person team of specialists to discuss all areas of chronic pain management in this 225-page workbook, $17.95 + $3.80 shipping and handling. New Harbinger Publications, Inc., 5674 Shattuck Avenue, Oakland, CA 94609; (800)748-6273.

Coping With Fibromyalgia by Beth Ediger and ***Fibromyalgia: Fighting Back*** by Bev Spencer, $6.95 each or $12.95 for two booklets (including postage). Prices for bulk orders on request. fax (416) 324-8850. LRH Publications, Box 8 Station Q, Toronto, Ontario M4T 2L7 Canada.

Examining Your Doctor by Timothy McCall, M.D. An excellent resource on evaluating the quality of your medical care, $16.95 + $4.00 shipping and handling. Carol Publishing Group, 120 Enterprise Avenue, Secaucus, NJ 07094; (800) 447-2665.

Fibromyalgia: A Comprehensive Approach by Miryam E. Williamson. 202-page source book of medical and non-medical strategies for relieving the agony of fibromyalgia, $14.95 + $3.75

shipping and handling. Walker and Company, 435 Hudson Street, New York, NY 10014; (800) 284-2553, fax (212) 727-0984.

Fibromyalgia and Chronic Myofascial Pain Syndrome: A Survival Manual by Devin Starlanyl, M.D., and Mary Ellen Copeland, M.S., M.A. This guide illustrates the differences between fibromyalgia and myofascial pain and discusses a variety of treatments, $19.95 + $3.80 shipping and handling. New Harbinger Publications, Inc., 5674 Shattuck Avenue, Oakland, CA 94609; (800) 748-6273.

The Fibromyalgia Helpbook by Jenny Fransen, R.N., and I. Jon Russell, M.D., Ph.D. 240-page how-to guide to living better with fibromyalgia, $18.95 + $4.00 shipping and handling. Order from Fransen and Associates, 1729 Lois Drive, Shoreview, MN 55126.

Fibromyalgia: Managing the Pain by Mark Pellegrino, M.D. 84-page comprehensive guide to fibromyalgia, $12.45 + $3.50 shipping and handling. Anadem Publishing, Inc., 3620 North High Street, Columbus, OH 43214; (800) 633-0055, fax (614) 262-6630.

The Fibromyalgia Supporter by Mark Pellegrino, M.D. A book for families of people with fibromyalgia with specific advice to help guide loved ones' responses to a variety of situations in day-to-day living, $15.50 + $3.50 shipping and handling. Anadem Publishing, Inc., 3620 North High Street, Columbus, OH 43214; (800) 633-0055, fax (614) 262-6630.

The Fibromyalgia Survivor by Mark Pellegrino, M.D. 120 pages of advice and tips on living your life to the fullest with fibromyalgia, $19.50 + $3.50 shipping and handling. Anadem Publishing, Inc., 3620 North High Street, Columbus, OH 43214; (800) 633-0055, fax (614) 262-6630.

The Fibromyalgia Syndrome by Mary Anne Saathoff, R.N. A booklet that describes fibromyalgia clearly and in depth, $4.00. Order from Fibromyalgia Alliance of America, P.O. Box 21990 Columbus, OH 43221-0990; (614) 457-4222, fax (614) 457-2729.

"Fibromyalgia Syndrome: An Informational Guide for FMS Patients, Their Families, Friends and Employers" (brochure) by Robert Bennett, M.D. FMS diagnosis, treatment, epidemiology, and exercise information. First one free with stamped envelope or 50 copies for $8.00. The National Fibromyalgia Research Assn., P.O. Box 500, Salem, OR 97308.

From Fatigued to Fantastic! by Jacob Teitelbaum, M.D. 183-page book by a physician who has experienced fibromyalgia and chronic fatigue syndrome and also treated patients with these conditions, $11.95 + $5.00 shipping and handling. Order from Jacob Teitelbaum, M.D., 466 Forelands Road, Annapolis, MD 21401; (800) 333-5287, fax (410) 266-6104.

Getting the Most Out of Your Medicines 54-page booklet that reviews the drugs available for FMS/CFIDS treatment, discusses why they might work and offers tips on how patients may receive the most benefits from them, $10.00. Order from Fibromyalgia Network, P.O. Box 3175, Tucson, AZ 85751-1750; (602) 290-5508, fax (602) 290-5550.

The Honest Herbal by Varro Tyler, Ph.D. This book is a good reference on herbal therapies, $17.95 + $4.00 shipping and handling. Haworth Medical Press, 10 Alice Street, Binghampton, NY 13904; (800) 429-6784, fax (800) 895-0582.

Laugh at Your Muscles by Mark Pelligrino, M.D. 92-page light read of humorous insights into fibromyalgia, $5.95 + $3.50 shipping and handling. Anadem Publishing, Inc., 3620 North High Street, Columbus, OH 43214; (800) 633-0055, fax (614) 262-6630.

Managing Pain Before It Manages You by Margaret A. Caudill, M.D., Ph.D. 207-page manual that discusses a variety of cognitive approaches to understanding and working with chronic pain, $18.95 + $4.00 shipping and handling. The Guildford Press, 72 Spring Street, New York, NY 10012; (800) 365-7006.

Running On Empty: The Complete Guide to Chronic Fatigue Syndrome by Katrina Berne, Ph.D. Written by a clinical psychologist who has CFIDS herself, with updated resources and guidelines for managing this condition, $14.95 + $2.50 shipping and handling. Hunter House Inc., P.O. Box 2914, Alameda, CA 94501-0914; (800) 266-5592, fax (510) 865-4295.

Sick and Tired of Being Sick and Tired - Living with Invisible Chronic Illness by Paul J. Donoghue, Ph.D., and Mary Siegel, Ph.D. 248-page book, $11.95+ $3.50 shipping and handling. W.W. Norton & Co., Dept. JWB, 500 5th Avenue, New York, NY 10110; (800) 233-4830.

Solving the Puzzle of CFIDS by Murray Susser, M.D., and Michael Rosenbaum, M.D. 170-page book, $28.00. Dr. Murray Susser, 2730 Wilshire Blvd. #110, Santa Monica, CA 94043.

Successful Living With Chronic Illness: Celebrating the Joys of Life by Kathleen Lewis. $14.95 + $4.00 shipping. Kendall/Hunt Publishing Co., 4050 Westmark Dr., P.O. Box 1840, Dubuque, IA 52004-1840.

TMJ: Its Many Faces by Wesley Shankland, D.D.S., M.S. 140-page comprehensive book for individuals with pain in the temporamandibular joint. Basic TMJ information is detailed along with specific treatment options, $19.50 + $3.50 shipping and handling. Anadem Publishing, Inc., 3620 North High Street, Columbus, OH 43214; (800) 633-0055, fax (614) 262-6630.

The Truth About TMJ: How to Help Yourself by Jennifer Hutchinson. 205-page book, $16.00. Order from Reinhardt & Still Publishers, Box 3232, Winchester, VA 22604; (800) 303-2244.

Understanding Post Traumatic Fibromyalgia by Mark J. Pellegrino, M.D. 122-page book that discusses the assessment, treatment and prognosis of fibromyalgia following a motor vehicle accident, work injury or other trauma, $16.25 + $3.50 shipping and handling. Anadem Publishing, Inc., 3620 North High Street, Columbus, OH 43214; (800) 633-0055, fax (614) 262-6630.

We Laughed, We Cried: Life With Fibromyalgia compiled and edited by Kit Gardiser and Kathleen Kerry. 177 pages of personal stories of people with fibromyalgia are expressed in poetry, prose, cartoons, sketches, drawings and photography, $13.50. KMK Associates, P.O. Box 60246, Palo Alto, CA 94306.

When Muscle Pain Won't Go Away: The Relief Handbook for Fibromyalgia and Chronic Muscle Pain by Gayle Backstrom with B.R. Rubin, DO, FACP, $15.95. Taylor Publishing Company, 1550 W. Mockingbird Lane, Dallas, TX 75235.

When You're Sick and Don't Know Why by Linda Hanner and John Witek, M.D. A 240-page book that discusses the trials of searching for a diagnosis, $12.95. DCI Publishing, P.O. Box 47945, Minneapolis, MN 55447; (800) 848-2793.

Disability Resources

How To Apply For Social Security Disability Benefits If You Have Chronic Fatigue Syndrome.
Massachusetts CFIDS Assn., 808 Main Street, Waltham, MA 02154; (617) 893-4415.

Social Security Disability Benefits: How To Get Them! How To Keep Them! James W. Ross,
R.D. 3, Three Forrester Road, Slippery Rock, PA 16057; (412) 794-2837.

Social Security Disability Benefits Information. Pamphlet, National Chronic Fatigue Syndrome
Assn., 3521 Broadway, Suite 222, Kansas City, MO 64111; (816) 931-4777.

Understanding Social Security and ***Disability Evaluation Under Social Security.*** Social Security
Administration, Baltimore, MD 21235; (800) 772-1213.

Educational Resources

Atlantic Regional Conference on Fibromyalgia, P.O. Box 22008, Lansdowne P.O., Saint John,
New Brunswick, Canada; (506) 634-2883, fax (506) 652-2305.

Fibromyalgia Educational Systems, Inc. - Publisher of this ***Taking Charge of Fibromyalgia***
handbook and also an educational program package to correspond with this handbook. The
program package includes a teaching manual, color slides and a patient handbook. The authors
have first-hand knowledge of fibromyalgia because they too live with this condition. For more
information, contact Fibromyalgia Educational Systems, 500 Bushaway Road, Wayzata, MN
55391; (612) 473-6218 or (419) 843-3153.

Health Catalog

Self Care - Helpful catalog which offers various self-care tools such as full spectrum lights for
treating seasonal affective disorder, thera canes, heated mattress pads, air filters, electric
massagers, vitamins, etc. No claims are made by FES for the efficacy of these products. Self
Care, 5850 Shellmound Street, Emeryville, CA 94608; (800) 345-3371, fax (800) 345-4021.

Internet Resources

There is a growing wealth of information on the Internet that offers the user a variety of advice,
opinions, research-based findings, resources, etc. on fibromyalgia. There are support groups, chat
rooms and even excerpts of newsletters and books available for you to peruse. Many
organizations, including ours, have websites for you to explore. We encourage you to show
healthy skepticism when using the Internet, since it does not have a mechanism for quality control.
Some of the information you find may be valid and some may not. Discuss new information you
discover on the Internet with professionals who are well informed on fibromyalgia. This step will
help you separate quality information from some that may be harmful to your health.

The following is a sampling of the websites available on fibromyalgia to help you start your search
on the worldwide web. A main source for information is found in alt.med.fibromyalgia.

Arthritis Foundation
http:/www.arthritis. org

Colorado Health Network
http://bcn.boulder.co.us/health/chn/fibro/fibro_center.html

Fibromyalgia Association of British Columbia Library
http://204.244.17.10/libs/hefibrom.htm

Fibromyalgia Educational Systems, Inc. (our site)
http.www. fmsedsys.com

Fibromyalgia Newsgroup
news:alt.med.fibromyalgia

Fibromyalgia Patient Support
http://www.fix.net/~esargent/fms

FMS Website on AOL
http://users.aol.com/fmswebpage/fmshome.html or
http://membrs.aol.com/fmswebpage/fmshome.html

Health Road Productions
http://pomo.nbn.com/people/healthrd

Missouri Arthritis Rehabilitation Research
http://www.hsc.missouri.edu/fibro

National Fibromyalgia Research Assn
http://www.teleport.com/~nfra/.teleport.com/~nfra/

Oregon Fibromyalgia Foundation
http://www.anawave.com/~OFF

Sapient Heatlh Network (SHN)
http://www.shn.net

Medical Journals

Journal of Musculoskeletal Pain—Peer-reviewed medical journal containing FMS scientific abstract information. Appropriate for lay people as well as medical professionals. Quarterly publication. Cost: $36.00 annual subscription. Haworth Medical Press, 10 Alice Street, Binghamton, NY 13904; (800) 342-9678, fax (800) 895-0582.

Journal of the Chronic Fatigue Syndrome—Peer-reviewed medical journal containing CFIDS scientific abstract information. Appropriate for lay people as well as medical professionals. Quarterly publication. Cost: $36.00 annual subscription. Haworth Medical Press, 10 Alice Street, Binghamton, NY 13904; (800) 342-9678, fax (800) 895-0582.

Newsletters

The CFIDS Chronicle - A quarterly publication aimed at reporting the most current CFIDS/FMS research information. Other publications available as well as information about the Association and member benefits. The CFIDS Assn. of America, Inc., PO Box 220398, Charlotte, NC 28222-0398; (800) 442-3437.

Fibromyalgia Frontiers - FMS quarterly membership publication of the Greater Washington, D.C., Fibromyalgia Assn. Information regarding FMS research advances, treatment ideas, conventions and advocacy issues. Cost: $18.00 annual membership fee. Fibromyalgia Frontiers, P.O. Box 2373, Centreville, VA 22020; (703) 790-2324.

Fibromyalgia Network - Kristin Thorson, FMS patient advocate, editor. Quarterly newsletter covering advances in FMS and CFIDS research as well as patient education, advocacy and convention information. Cost: $19.00 for annual subscription in U.S. and $21.00 U.S. funds for Canadian residents. Fibromyalgia Network Newsletter, P.O. Box 3175, Tucson, AZ 85751-1750; (800) 853-2929, fax (520) 290-5550.

Fibromyalgia Alliance of America Newsletter - A quarterly publication, Mary Anne Saathoff, R.N., FMS patient and editor. Addresses FMS coping strategies as well as up-to-date research and treatment advances, videos and conference information. Cost: $25.00 yearly in U.S., $30.00 in Canada, and $35.00 international. Fibromyalgia Alliance of America, P.O. Box 21990, Columbus, OH 43221-0990; (614) 457-4222, fax (614) 457-2729.

From Fatigued to Fantastic Newsletter - Jacob Teitelbaum, M.D. Cost: $29.95 for 3 issues/year. Jacob Teitelbaum, M.D., 466 Forelands Road, Annapolis, MD 21401; (800) 333-5287, fax (410) 266-6104.

Inspire Newsletter - A newsletter for women with a chronic illness. Cost: $15.00 for 6 issues/year in U.S., $18.00 U.S. funds for Canadian residents, $22.00 elsewhere. Inspire Newsletter, P.O. Box 081553, Racine, WI 53408-1553; (414) 639-7745.

Seattle FMS Association Newsletter - A quarterly publication. Fibromyalgia International Team, Inc., P.O. Box 77373, Seattle, WA 98177-0373; phone/fax (206) 362-2310.

Organizations

Arthritis Foundation - Publishes and distributes FMS pamphlets and brochures, as well as other printed information regarding rheumatoid and osteo arthritis, Lupus, and other illnesses. Chapters located in many U.S. cities and towns. Also offers a self-help class in some communities; contact your local chapter.

The CFIDS Organization of America, Inc. - Includes a newsletter, resources, discounts in their buying club for prescriptions and nutritional supplements. Annual membership - $35.00. The CFIDS Organization of America, Inc., P.O. Box 220398, Charlotte, NC 28222-0398; (800) 442-3437, fax (704) 365-9755.

Fibromyalgia Alliance of America - Includes quarterly newsletter (refer to newsletter section for detailed description). Mary Anne Saathoff, R.N., president and FMS patient. P.O. Box 21990, Columbus, OH 43221-0990; (614) 457-4222, fax (614) 457-2729. Membership fees: $25.00 yearly in U.S., $30.00 in Canada, and $35.00 international.

FMS Support Groups - Many U.S. and Canadian cities have active FMS support groups. For information, call your hospital, state chapter of the Arthritis Foundation or The Fibromyalgia Network, P.O. Box 3175, Tucson, AZ 85751-1750; (800) 853-2929, fax (520) 290-5550.

National Fibromyalgia Research Association. - A nonprofit organization dedicated to education, treatment and finding a cure for FMS. NFRA funds research, supplies educational materials to physicians and helps raise FMS public awareness. National Fibromyalgia Research Assn., P.O. Box 500, Salem, OR 97308; (503) 588-1411 ext. 2265. Rae Gleason, activist.

Pharmacies for Special Prescriptions

Belmar Pharmacy, Lakewood, CO (800) 525-9473.

Professional Arts Pharmacy (800) 832-9285.

Women's International Pharmacy, Madison, WI (800) 279-5708.

Videos

Fibromyalgia Exercise. Video by Patty Bourne, Kinesiologist - Excellent 30-minute video illustrating correct FMS exercise regimen - $24.50. OTM Hospital, Physiology Dept., 327 Reynolds Street, Oakville, Ontario L6J 3L7, Canada.

Fibromyalgia: Face to Face. 14-minute insight into living with FMS from people, including children, who are coping with this syndrome. Also features three prominent FMS research doctors - $19.95. Ontario Fibromyalgia Assn., 250 Cloor Street East, Suite 902, Toronto, Ontario M4W 3P2, Canada.

Fibromyalgia and You. Video by I. Jon Russell, M.D., PhD. 90 minutes of up-to-date information on all aspects of fibromyalgia. It features various fibromyalgia researchers and physicians and five patients who describe their stories - $34.95. Fibromyalgia Information Resources, P.O. Box 690402, San Antonio, TX 78269.

Fibromyalgia: What Do We Know. 30-minute video on coping with FMS as described by patients who are successfully managing their illness. Reviews sleep disorders, treatment, medications, exercise, stress management and other pain remedies - $19.95. FM Association of B.C., P.O. Box 15455, Vancouver, B.C. V6B 5B2, Canada.

Manual Tender Point Survey. 15-minute video for physicians to illustrate the correct method of performing this important diagnostic exam - $10.00. Make check out to University Anesthesia and Critical Care Medicine Foundation and send to Pain Evaluation and Treatment Institute, 4601 Baum Boulevard, Pittsburgh, PA 15213-1217, (412) 578-3100.

Stretching: Fibromyalgia Exercise Video. 36-minute video includes an explanation by Dr. Sharon Clark of why stretching is so important for people with fibromyalgia and a demonstration featuring individuals with FMS - $24.95. Order from Oregon Fibromyalgia Foundation, 1221 S.W. Yamhill, Suite 303, Portland, OR 97205. Dr. Clark is in the process of developing a strengthening video for people with fibromyalgia. When completed, it will be available at the Oregon Fibromyalgia Foundation.

Vitamin Testing

Vitamin Diagnostics, Cliffwood Beach, New Jersey (908) 583-7773.

Alternative Care Resource List

American Association of Naturopathic
Physicians
2366 Eastlake Avenue East
Seattle, WA 98102
206-323-7610
fax: 206-323-7612

American Botanical Council
PO Box 201660
Austin, TX 78720-1660
513-331-8868

American Chiropractic Association
1701 Clarendon Blvd.
Arlington, VA 22209
800-986-4636

American Herbalists Guild
Box 1683
Soquel, CA 95073
408-438-1700

American Holistic Medical Association
4101 Lake Boone Trail, Ste. 201
Raleigh, NC 27607
919-787-5181

American Holistic Nurses Association
4101 Lake Boone Trail, Ste. 201
Raleigh, NC 27607
919-787-5181

American Massage Therapy Associaton
820 Davis Street, Ste. 100
Evanston, IL 60201
708-864-0123

American Osteopathic Association
142 East Ontario Street
Chicago, IL 60611
312-280-5800

American Society of Clinical Hypnosis
2200 East Devon Avenue, Ste. 291
Des Plaines, IL 60018
847-297-3317

Association for Applied
Psychophysiology and Biofeedback
10200 West 44th Avenue, Ste. 304
Wheat Ridge, CO 80033
303-422-8436
fax: 303-422-8894

Biofeedback Certification Association
10200 West 44th Avenue, Ste. 304
Wheat Ridge, CO 80033
303-420-2902
fax: 303-422-8894

National Center for Homeopathy
801 North Fairfax Street, Ste. 306
Alexandria, VA 22314
703-548-7790

National Commission for the
Certification of Acupuncturists
1424 16th Street N.W., Ste. 501
Washington, DC 20036
202-232-1404

RESOURCES

FREE Health Catalog & Newspaper

To Your Health, Inc.

To Your Health, Inc., is a family-based company offering natural health products for those with fibromyalgia, chronic fatigue, arthritis and chronic pain. The products are featured in two publications, a catalog and newspaper, and both are *free* for the asking.

David and Margret Squires, the co-founders of **To Your Health, Inc.,** are in the business for very personal reasons. David has had fibromyalgia for 30 years. Both publications feature his story of how he searched for a diagnosis, treatment, and information about fibromyalgia (FMS). What he found was that natural therapy in both nutrition and treatment were the most beneficial for him. Not wishing others to go through what he did, he wanted to provide a resource so others would not face the same frustrations in dealing with FMS. David and Margret founded **To Your Health, Inc.,** in July of 1994, with only 8 products in their resource catalog. A year later, they published their second catalog with over 35 products (adding several good health tools of books, tapes, and therapeutic devices) and launched a resource newspaper as well. Their company is dedicated to the cause of raising awareness and providing education about FMS, CFIDS, arthritis, and chronic pain.

Their *Resource Catalog* features vitamins and health products developed specifically to help these chronic conditions. One product in particular shown by researchers to help fibromyalgia is a magnesium and malic acid combination found in the company's product, Fibro-Care™. Another product which helps in all chronic pain conditions is Pain Control Formula™, an aloe-based lotion with capsaicin, which reduces substance-P, a neurotransmitter of pain. An explanation of each product and why it was chosen is included in the catalog. In *Health • Points, a Resource Newspaper for those with FMS, CFIDS, Arthritis, and Chronic Pain,* they include all the products of the catalog but also feature articles of interest such as finding appropriate complementary and medical treatment, pain management, nutrition, and physical therapy, written by caring health professionals who are knowledgeable about FMS, CFIDS, arthritis, and chronic pain.

FOR YOUR FREE COPY: For a copy of either the catalog or the newspaper, call (800) 801-1406, *OR* send a postcard to: **To Your Health, Inc.,** 11809 Nightingale Circle, Fountain Hills, AZ 85268.

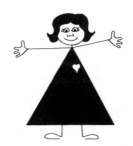

Appendix: Physician Protocols

Treatment of Fibromyalgia and Chronic Fatigue Syndrome Using The Oxytocin-Hormonal-Nutrient Protocol

by Jorge D. Flechas, M.D., M.P.H.

Dr. Flechas is a family practitioner in North Carolina who works with patients who have fibromyalgia syndrome (FMS) and patients with chronic fatigue and immune dysfunction syndrome (CFIDS). He has developed a new protocol for treatment of these illnesses using oxytocin (OT), dehydroepiandrosterone (DHEA) and some natural nutrients. He feels both diseases are most likely due to a neuroendocrine/metabolic disorder with chronic hypoxia, which causes abnormalities in the biochemistry of patients.

This summary of information is divided into two sections. Section I contains the technical perspective and Section II the treatment plan. Some readers may wish to review the treatment plan for its applicability to their situation and then become familiar with the technical perspective.

Section I: Medical Perspective

FMS and CFIDS are different diseases but closely related. Patients with these diseases have in common a decrease in corticotrophin releasing hormone (CRH), which controls cortisol output from the adrenals.[1-4] Both groups of patients have shown a decrease in levels of arginine vasopressin (AVP), a hormone that controls the ability of the body to release fluid.[1,2,5] With a lack of this hormone patients feel increasingly thirsty and have frequent urination, about every 20 to 30 minutes. Both of these hormones are produced in an area of the brain called the supraoptic nucleus. Another hormone of importance, called oxytocin (OT), is produced by the same nerve cells. The same neurons that make OT also have the capacity of making CRH and AVP.[6] As of October of 1997, no one in the medical literature had described an OT deficiency. An attempt to define an OT deficiency will be done here.

Oxytocin

OT is a hormone produced in many parts of the body. In the brain, it is produced and released on a daily rhythm with its peak occurring at around noon.[7,8] OT is also produced in the posterior retina, in the pineal gland, thymus, pancreas, testicle, ovary, and adrenal glands. Oxytocin's known functions will be discussed below.

1. OT is known to control the microcirculation of the human body and brain.[9-12] A decrease in OT can cause problems with decreased circulation in the extremities. Therefore, patients often complain of cold hands and feet, along with a history of recurrent headaches. Oxytocin's ability to vasodilate the blood vessels is due to its capacity to stimulate the body's cells to produce nitric oxide, a powerful vasodilator of microcirculation.[9-11] If vasodilation, such as blushing, does not occur when OT is given intramuscularly, then a serious defect in nitric oxide production is present. This defect of poor circulation is often present among FMS/CFIDS patients.[13-15]

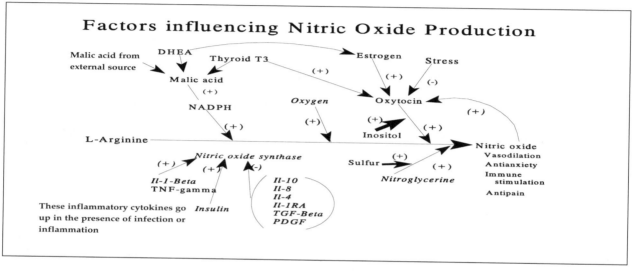

2. OT is released as a mother nurses her baby.[16] Stimulation of the hormone release causes the mother to have an instinct to want to cuddle. As she nurses the child, her desire to cuddle intensifies. This same feeling can be experienced during intimacy–OT has the ability to increase libido.[17,18] Therefore, patients lacking this hormone may often notice that they do not wish to cuddle, to be held, or to be intimate. It has been noticed that stress can restrain the production of OT.[19-21]

3. OT seems to stimulate the ability of the brain to concentrate, contribute to mental alertness, and improve memory. [22] Patients lacking this hormone may find difficulty in concentrating and feel like they are thinking in a fog. This has been noted in FMS.[23-25]

4. OT can occupy multiple hormonal receptor sites in the body. Dr. Flechas theorizes that an empty receptor for OT can potentially cause pain. Administering OT causes the empty OT receptor sites to become full, thereby diminishing or completely obliterating pain. Animal studies reveal that because of this particular characteristic, OT has been an effective tool in weaning addicted animals from narcotics, suggesting that OT has the ability to occupy not only its own receptor sites, but opiate (narcotic) receptor sites as well.[26]

5. OT is produced in the posterior retina of the eye.[27] A decrease in OT level can cause problems with intermittent blurring of vision. When OT is given, it can sharpen the vision. (clinical observation) In patients with reduced levels of OT, one can expect complaints of pain in the posterior eye, sometime so severe that only narcotics provide effective pain relief. Visual disturbances in FMS have been observed.[28,29]

6. OT is also made in the pineal gland of the brain, as is melatonin, a hormone which enhances sleep.[27,30] In animal studies, as the level of OT increases in the brain, the animal is induced into a deeper sleep.[30] (Insomnia is a sleep disorder frequently seen in patients with FMS/CFIDS, and could indicate a deficiency in melatonin.) Note: Recent research indicates that melatonin has the ability to activate the immune system, so the use of this product is usually contraindicated in the presence of autoimmune disease (such as lupus, rheumatoid arthritis).[31]

7. The ovaries make OT.[32,33] In the ovary, OT helps in the fine-tuning of progesterone release.[32] When patients are lacking OT, they may frequently complain of ovarian pain, even though pathology does not support the presence of either cysts or tumors. Ovulation function may be impaired with menstrual irregularity.[28]

8. OT is synthesized in the adrenal glands where it stimulates or inhibits steroid production.[21,34-37] Patients with decreased OT levels often complain of flank pain underneath the posterior ribs. Malfunction in the adrenal steroid production has been seen in FMS.[38,39]

9. OT is created by the thymus gland.[40,41] The thymus gland utilizes OT to help process white blood cells which help control autoimmunity. Normal levels of OT also help stimulate these cells into greater action.[40-46] For example, it is a known fact that women who nurse their children have a much lesser incidence of breast cancer. This hormone may be protective in its ability to prevent breast cancer, through its influences on the immune system.[47]

10. OT is produced by the pancreas.[48] In the pancreas, OT is known to stimulate the production of glucagon, a hormone which helps the intestines to relax.[49,50] Therefore, in treating a patient with decreased levels of this hormone, one would expect to see problems with increased intestinal spasms, secondary to a lack of glucagon production from the pancreas.

11. OT can function as an antianxiety agent in the brain. It can also stimulate social behavior.[51] A lack of this hormone may be expressed as antisocial behavior with some anxiety.

12. OT can function as an antidepressant.[52] In low levels of OT one would expect to see depression, which has been noticed in FMS/CFIDS.[24,53]

13. OT can serve as a regulator of cardiovascular and autonomic nervous system function.[54,55] This explains why patients lacking this hormone have trouble controlling their blood pressure when going from a sitting to upright position, or when standing for a long period of time This is known as neurally mediated hypotension. They often complain of near syncope (light headed) and possible dizziness.[28] OT is found in the sections of the brain where the baroreceptors of the body are controlled.[55] A drop of OT levels in the brain leads to a manifestation of baroreceptor malfunction. Restoration of OT as an oral tablet (Belmar Pharmacy) corrects the symptoms of neurally mediated hypotension. (clinical observation)

14. OT has the capacity to induce the body to mildly retain fluid. This is in part due to its physical and biological similarity to arginine vasopressin.[11,56,57] AVP is a hormone that controls fluid metabolism and memory.[1,2,5] With a lack of OT, patients have increased thirst. They also have increased urinary output due to decreased ability to retain fluid.[28]

As can be seen, the actions and normal functions which have been associated with the use of OT are broad and varied. The following diagram helps to illustrate and contrast the known functions of OT

Other Symptoms/Syndromes Associated with Fibromyalgia	Functions of Oxytocin
Cognitive difficulties: memory loss, decreased concentration, depression Headaches Numbness or tingling Eye complaints Vestibular complaints: dizziness, vertigo Temporomandibular joint syndrome (TMJ) Esophageal dysmotility Mitral valve prolapse: heart palpitations, chest pain (non-cardiac) Lung symptoms Joint hypermobility Irritable bowel syndrome Painful menstruation Interstitial cystitis Vulvodynia: painful sexual intercourse Vestibulitis Female urethral syndrome Multiple chemical hypersensitivity Painful arches of the feet Microcirculation disturbances: cold hands and feet	Increased alertness, concentration, and desire to cuddle Improves and restores memory Combats depression Promotes clear vision Stabilizes neurological control of blood pressure Enhances fluid retention Enhances sleep and relaxation Enhances microcirculation of hands, feet and head Helps to control pain in muscles and joints Stimulates or inhibits steroid production in the body Helps bowels to relax Increases thermogenesis (body warmth) Stimulates lactation Stimulates labor in childbirth Improves sperm function Plays an important role in achieving orgasm Fine tunes progesterone production from ovary

and other symptoms of FMS, which are not commonly known in the regular medical literature.

Dehydroepiandrosterone

In treating FMS/CFIDS patients, a hormone of importance is dehydroepiandrosterone (DHEA). The adrenal glands produce between 30 and 50 mg. of DHEA per day, as compared to 10 mg. of cortisol. Hence, the major steroid released by the adrenals is DHEA. DHEA sulfate is the water-soluble form of the hormone inside the body. DHEA is a waxy substance and is very difficult for the body to transport from the adrenals to the tissues. Therefore, by sulfating the hormone, the body makes it water soluble and easier to transport to the respective tissues that need it. The following paragraphs, one through eleven, explore the physiologic functions of DHEA.

1. DHEA is the primary steroid produced when a baby is in utero.[67,68] At that time, the level of DHEA in the fetus is around 200 mcg./dl. At birth, DHEA levels drop considerably within a period of two to three weeks and will not significantly rise again until the age of 7. The hormone will continue to rise until the age of 25 in males and 32 in females. From these ages on, DHEA levels start dropping, and by age 60 to 70, will be 5 to 10 percent of the hormone level of a normal person 30 years old.[69]

2. DHEA assists in the production of oil in the human skin, as does thyroid and betacarotene. When DHEA is lacking, the skin becomes dry and rough.[70] Patients with low DHEA levels find themselves constantly applying lotion. DHEA also helps to control all hair production in the female, from her head to her toes. A woman experiencing a low level of DHEA will notice a

APPENDIX

decrease in hair production on the legs, underarms and pubic area and some loss of hair on top of the head. Sometime women will simply notice a need to shave less often. Some patients report that DHEA therapy has helped to increase oil production in their hair. Patients on DHEA hormonal replacement therapy have also noticed that skin and nails begin to get thicker, hair becomes less gray, grows faster, and becomes more dense. Smoother, younger looking skin has been an additional benefit that many patients find attractive while taking DHEA.

3. DHEA helps to maintain skeletal mass. Therefore, patients with a decrease in DHEA will have accelerated problems with loss of bone mass.[71,72]

4. DHEA can stimulate the immune system.[73-78] Therefore, with low DHEA, problems with increased infections are noted. In addition, a person with low levels of DHEA requires a longer period of time to recover from a cold and other illnesses, as compared to normal individuals. The steroid also declines with aging.[79]

As mentioned earlier, DHEA is the primary steroid produced by the human adrenal glands.[69] When the body undergoes inflammation from infection or surgical stress, the production of DHEA drops and the adrenal cortisol output increases.[80,81] This process is known in the medical literature as adrenal adaptation syndrome.[80] Chronic inflammation, as seen in lupus, rheumatoid arthritis, tuberculosis, or any long-term infection, is not in the best interest of the body. Overcoming infection when the adrenals are functioning properly is much easier and accomplished in much less time than it is when the immune system is compromised with constant inflammation persisting.

DHEA can override cortisol's immunosuppressive effects on the immune system. One chemical pathway by which DHEA accomplishes this is by reversal of cortisol inhibition of the synthesis and secretion of gamma interferon.[82] Gamma interferon is a hormone produced by white blood cells to help stimulate the immune system to be involved in the protection of the body against infection, as seen in a viral infection.

DHEA is known to inhibit the cellular transformation of Epstein-Barr herpes virus, the virus known to cause mononucleosis.[83,84] When the human body has plenty of DHEA, the immune system is able to control the mononucleosis virus more effectively. When DHEA is low, one would then expect to see reactivation of not only the mononucleosis virus, but possibly other herpetic viruses potentially leading toward a syndrome known as latent herpes virus reactivation phenomena. This would help to explain why patients with CFIDS and FMS may have reoccurrences of herpetic infections such as genital herpes, cold sores, and shingles. Shingles is a reactivation of the chicken pox virus, a known herpes virus.

Patients with AIDS who have low levels of DHEA have been noted in medical studies to die sooner than those with higher levels of DHEA.[85] It appears that an AIDS patient with a higher level of DHEA presents a challenge to the HIV virus.

In laboratory studies, animals given an intentionally lethal dose of a virus predictably died.[85] In these same studies, animals given DHEA a few hours before receiving the "lethal dose" of a virus injection have been shown to survive. This demonstrates DHEA's ability to help the body resist viral infection.

DHEA can increase the size of the spleen germinal centers suggesting stimulation of the B-Lymphocyte dependant areas of the immune system. These cells are responsible for antibody production.[86] DHEA helps in the antibody conversion of IgM to IgG.[75] One of the major antibodies produced by the B-Lymphocyte(s) of the immune system is the IgM antibody. This is a large molecule that needs to be separated to make the IgG antibody. It is felt by some that to separate the IgM molecule into IgG is controlled by DHEA.

Studies performed indicate that DHEA acts as an anti-cancer steroid.[83,87-89] Low levels of DHEA are associated with an increase in breast cancer, bladder, gastric, and prostate cancer.[90-94] A cancer diagnosis could imply that a low level of DHEA probably existed prior to the time of diagnosis.

5. The ability to detoxify chemicals is controlled by the liver. Drugs and other foreign substances in our bodies, such as silicone, antibiotics and other drugs, are referred to as xenobiotics. Metabolism, or detoxification of these xenobiotics, takes place via two different major pathways: Phase I (oxidation) and Phase II (conjugation).

Phase I occurs inside the cell, while Phase II occurs in the liver. It is possible to measure both of these operations to determine whether each is functioning properly. It is not only possible to determine if a patient is suffering from chemical overload, but also to identify which part of the detoxification pathway is damaged. Common problems presenting a chemically sensitive patient are that one or both of the processes are overworked or depleted. This is important so that appropriate nutrient therapy can begin repairing the affected injured pathway.

Testing can also identify whether exposure to chemicals is causing cellular damage and other disease symptoms. Measurements can be taken after a few days at home, then repeated after a few days at work. Using this approach can help to establish which environment is more damaging to the detoxification pathways.

According to experts, most patients suffering from a major illness would exhibit a low level of DHEA if tested. Unfortunately, these untested, chronically ill patients are often the very ones who are investigating detoxification as a potential approach to improve overall health. Experts fear that those initiating a detoxification program with a low DHEA level could potentially place more stress on an already burdened liver. This would in turn prolong the detoxification process and possibly threaten the well-being of the patient.

On the other hand, initiating such a program once the DHEA level is higher could offer the participant less discomfort throughout the detoxification period, as it is known that DHEA has demonstrated the ability to stimulate the Phase II (liver) detoxification process and also assist in Phase I detoxification.[95,96]

Patients receiving DHEA therapy experience less sensitivity to medications. Patients frequently find that they are able to tolerate both increasing the dosage of existing medications and adding additional medications. Clinical observation has suggested that once DHEA therapy is in place, the patient is able to detoxify drugs and other chemicals effectively, as the body approaches a normal detoxification process.

6. DHEA has unique properties that are responsible for the ways it interacts with itself. DHEA has no feedback on itself.[97] There is no documented evidence of DHEA production being inhibited with hormonal replacement therapy of DHEA.[98] It is known that the self-production of thyroid greatly decreases when patients are given oral thyroid hormone. This same principle holds

true for the administration of cortisol; the adrenal gland slows production of cortisol when a patient receives cortisol preparations.

DHEA also has unique functions when interacting with other hormones. The active hormone produced by the thyroid is a hormone called thyroid T3. Although DHEA has no direct effect on the T3 levels of the body, recently it has been shown that DHEA works to potentiate the active free T3 function, making it more effective in its work at the cellular level.[99]

In diabetes, it has been noted that DHEA helps to enhance insulin binding to its receptors on the cell membrane and also to its action on cells.[100,101]

It is felt that DHEA is the main hormone which helps to control the female libido.[102] Most female sex steroid hormones are dependent on DHEA for their existence.[102] Therefore, DHEA controls the production of estrogens and androgens (male hormones). This can potentially influence fertility, libido, and improve PMS. (Clinical observation)

7. Inside each cell of the body are approximately 800 mitochondria which help produce energy for the cells. This energy can be used by cells for normal cellular function or be used to help heat the body. The process of heating the human body is called thermogenesis. It has been shown that when DHEA is given, thermogenesis increases.[103] Patients receiving oral DHEA therapy report feeling warmer.

Inside the mitochondria, DNA is present and helps to produce some of the enzymes inside the mitochondria. DHEA is known to stimulate the DNA production of these enzymes.[104,105] DHEA has been shown to increase basal oxygen consumption.[99] The hormone, when added to thyroid T3, has been shown to be helpful in activation of the malic enzyme gene transcription inside the mitochondria.[104] Overall, DHEA and thyroid T3 interact synergistically to stimulate the body to have more energy via the cellular mitochondria.

8. In human studies DHEA has been used in the treatment of cirrhosis,[106-108] psoriasis (as a topical solution),[109-112] lupus,[113] hereditary angioneurotic edema,[114] arteriosclerotic heart disease,[115] AIDS,[84] porphyria,[116] and has been shown to increase natural killer cells cytotoxicity.[117] DHEA has now been used in the treatments of disease such as multiple sclerosis,[118,119] post-menopausal depression,[120] and gout.[120] Clinically, it has been successfully used to treat a patient with porphyria. The patient could not tolerate five minutes of sunshine. When exposed to the sun, her skin would develop blisters and cause her to have severe itching. Within one month of hormonal replacement therapy with oral DHEA, she was able to be in the Florida sunshine for greater than eight hours per day with no reaction to the sun.

In the presence of DHEA, natural killer cells of the immune system are able to kill cancer cells and yeast cells more effectively. Clinically, it has been noted that yeast infections come under better control with less recurrences in the presence of taking DHEA. The overall number of natural killer cells is increased in the presence of DHEA.[117]

9. DHEA has been shown to be an anti-aging hormone. Clinical observations show that patients who have high levels of this hormone suffer less from the ravages of aging as compared to those who have lesser amounts of this hormone.[96]

10. DHEA has recently been shown to stimulate the production of serotonin, a chemical used by

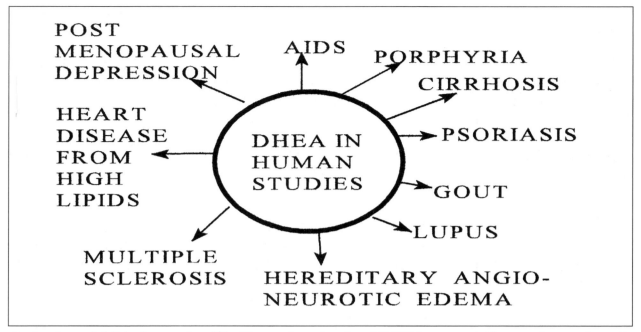

POST MENOPAUSAL DEPRESSION

AIDS

PORPHYRIA

CIRRHOSIS

HEART DISEASE FROM HIGH LIPIDS

DHEA IN HUMAN STUDIES

PSORIASIS

GOUT

LUPUS

MULTIPLE SCLEROSIS

HEREDITARY ANGIO-NEUROTIC EDEMA

the brain to inhibit depression.[121] Hence, low levels of DHEA can manifest as depression. In FMS, plasma serotonin levels have been found to be low.[122-124]

11. In recent medical literature, Dr. I. Jon Russell, a prominent FMS researcher, and others have shown that patients with FMS have much lower levels of DHEA sulfate as compared to normal patients.[38,39]

The relationship between Oxytocin and DHEA

OT travels to its receptor sites in certain cell membranes of the body, binds, and activates a chemical messenger called cyclic AMP (cAMP).[32] This cAMP creates a signal which moves through the cell membrane directly into the cell, then activates the inositol triphosphate system. Research literature supports that this inositol phosphate system is DHEA dependent and necessary for optimum OT function.[125] When this system is activated, the cells of the body are free to do the jobs they are designed to perform. OT acts much like a fine tuner, enhancing the functions which the body is already performing on its own.

Inositol

Inositol is a substance found in the liver, kidneys, skeletal and heart muscle, and is part of the vitamin B complex. Its highest levels are found in the brain.[126,127] In nature it is found in brown rice, vegetables and fruit. The activity of cells throughout the body is governed by an intricate network of signaling systems which translate outside information into internal signals, or second messengers. Inositol acts as a signal enhancer to transduct many cellular processes, such as secretion, metabolism, cell growth, and neurotransmission of light.[128-132] Inositol in a cell helps to increase cellular calcium. This helps the cell perform functions such as contract, produce a hormone, etc. Secondary messengers, or signal transductors, are important because it is thought that an imbalance of these messengers may be at least partially responsible for normal cells converting into cancerous ones. This system is also responsible for the ability of a cell to produce nitric oxide.[133]

At this point it is important to recognize that other natural chemicals have been found to enhance the human body's response to OT and DHEA. These are choline, malic acid, magnesium, creatine and thyroid T3.

Choline

This nutrient is involved in protein, fat, and normal carbohydrate metabolism. Its highest concentration in nature is found in the soybean. Although phosphatidyl choline (PC) is a natural component of every single membrane, it plays an especially notable role in supporting the membranes responsible for making energy, detoxifying chemicals, and preventing cancer. Dysfunction within the membranes of the body produces allergies, hormone dysregulation, and disease. A deficiency in this essential nutrient can slow the improvement or recovery phase of an illness, produce gradual memory loss, and encourage chemical over-sensitivity. Studies indicate the use of this nutrient in combination with others has been successful in slowing down some early cases of Alzheimer's Disease.

Diets are usually lacking in sufficient quantities of choline, as well as other nutrients needed for metabolism of PC. Successful PC treatment requires careful balancing with these other nutrients necessary for assimilation into body chemistry. Experts describe this nutrient's potential for healing as phenomenal because the effects of a satisfactory level are so far-reaching.

As the body detoxifies chemicals, even more phosphatidyl choline is needed, especially since our modern world exposes us to so many chemicals. If one part of the body is lacking sufficient PC to perform its job, it will simply borrow from another area. For example, if the body's liver needs more and elects to borrow from the brain, the brain becomes deficient in this substance and can produce mood swings and poor memory. The components necessary for building PC are also necessary for forming acetylcholine, which is the main neurotransmitter of the brain and a potent stimulator of nitric oxide production.[134,135] Correcting a PC deficiency often produces marked improvement in short-term memory, as well as in overall health.

According to nutritional experts, a dosage which supplies approximately 3 gm. of phosphatidyl choline is preferred. This dosage is sufficient to increase the choline levels in the brain by 50%; 9 gm. can actually double the brain's choline level. However, manufacturers are constantly changing formulations and diluting the product to become more cost effective, so finding the appropriate dosage can be a challenge.

Malic Acid

Malic acid is a valuable adjunct to this therapy because it plays an essential role in sugar metabolism and in the formation of ATP, the energy currency for physical activity and other important body functions. The energy we use to perform physical and mental tasks as well as to maintain normal function of the organs in our body comes from food product combustion after digestion. Energy comes from these combusted, digested food products combined with oxygen. This energy is stored as ATP for future use. ATP production requires magnesium, oxygen, phosphates, and oxygen. Conditions such as hypoxia (reduced oxygen supply) can lower ATP production. Further, conditions such as lower than optimal levels of magnesium, phosphate, and substrates will literally "shut down" the complete utilization of sugar for the manufacture of ATP.

As a result, the body will then switch to a very inefficient system of generating ATP. This involves the breaking down of proteins in muscles and other tissues. This is harmful to the body in the long run, resulting in damage to the affected parts. Physical symptoms usually associated with this breakdown are pain, decreased function, and fatigue. ATP levels have been found low in FMS.[136,137]

When OT levels are low, the cells of the body go into a state of hypoxia. This happens because OT via nitric oxide acts as a vasodilator to the capillaries. A lack of OT can potentially cause blood vessels to spasm, creating vicious cycles of more spasms which worsens the condition. It also further decreases the oxygen supply and food substances needed for ATP production. Malic acid is unique in its ability to increase the utilization of substances needed for ATP synthesis, and also has oxygen-sparing effects because it is able to generate ATP effectively by using sugar as fuel, even under low-oxygen conditions. This increase of ATP production under hypoxic conditions actually reverses blood vessel spasms and increases the amount of oxygen and food substances available to muscles and other tissues. Malic acid has also found uses in the treatment of liver disease because of its ability to eliminate ammonia, a substance very toxic to the brain. There are no known contraindications for the use of malic acid.[138]

Magnesium

In addition to malic acid, the other major player is magnesium, the fourth most abundant mineral in the body, and the second most abundant in muscles and organs. Magnesium is required for normal activity of 300 enzymes, including those involved in energy transfer from food to ATP and for transfer of energy from ATP to physical and mental activity. ATP forms a complex with magnesium, in order to stabilize the ATP molecule. An inadequate supply of magnesium can inhibit this process of energy production and the stability of its major energy component, ATP.[138] Magnesium insufficiency has presently been documented in both FMS/CFIDS.[138-140]

Creatine

Both FMS/CFIDS patients have low levels of creatine phosphate.[141-143] In the body creatine is used as a chemical to store energy. It can also serve as a major fuel for normal brain metabolism and as a stimulant for muscle building.[144-146]

Thyroid T3

The thyroid produces two major hormones, T4 and T3. Thyroid T4 will be absorbed in certain cells of the body where it is converted into T3. Many cells, such as liver, heart, skeletal muscles, and kidney cells, do not have the ability to convert T4 into T3 and must absorb T3 directly from the plasma. Thyroid T3 does its work in the DNA of the nucleus and of the mitochondria. The conversion of T4 to T3 will decrease under certain conditions. Some factors are aging, infection, inflammation, selenium deficiency, massive weight loss, fasting, and drugs.[147-153] When the thyroid T4 blood level is normal and the free T3 blood level is low, this is called Euthyroid Sick Syndrome.[154] FMS has been associated with hypothyroidism (low thyroid).[155-157]

How Are DHEA, T3, Malic Acid, Magnesium, Choline, Inositol, and Oxytocin Related?

The production of oxytocin and nitric oxide are dependant upon those substances below them in the following pyramid.

Both
Oxytocin and
Nitric Oxide function
best when these other hormones,
natural nutrients and minerals are present

Oxytocin	Nitric Oxide

Malic Acid	Choline	Inositol	Sulfur	Magnesium

Thyroid T3	Dehydroepianodrosterone (DHEA)

Section II: Treatment Plan

Understanding that the true success of any approach to treatment lies in the ability to reach patients outside the parameters of a single medical practice, a protocol has been developed for other treating physicians, using the aforementioned preparations. Double-blind, placebo-controlled testing of these hormones and nutrients has not been performed because of lack of funding. The clinician may wish to try them sequentially in individual patients.

First Office Visit

During this visit the diagnosis is made of a patient's medical problem. Lab work is done to get a baseline on the patient. Thyroid T3 and DHEA sulfate blood levels are measured on all FMS/CFIDS patients. The recommendations of DHEA researchers is that the blood levels of both male and female patients should be around 200 mcg. per dl. or greater. If the DHEA sulfate level is lower in a patient, then he or she is started on hormonal replacement therapy with DHEA. If the patient does not respond to the OT test dose with facial flushing and redness of the ears, then he or she is placed on DHEA in the A.M. for three months. If the DHEA-S04 value is below 200 mcg./dl., a good starting point is to begin treatment with DHEA 25 mg. p.o. (by mouth), every morning. DHEA converts to DHEA-S04 in the liver and is a stable hormone; a steady state exists between DHEA and DHEA-SO4. Therefore, treatment with DHEA-SO4 would not be of value. Please see below for dosage based on blood levels.

Recent work on neurosteroids from the brain has shown that DHEA in some patients may be excitatory to the brain. Hence, if one experiences problems with insomnia with DHEA, then the hormone should be taken in the morning. DHEA stimulates the DNA of the cells to produce the enzymes of the inositol triphosphate system. This allows the cells to be more reactive to OT stimulation when it occurs. This increase in reactivity of cells to OT may take up to three months to become fully operational. An easy way to probe this reactivity is by giving a patient a test dose of OT 10 units IM in the office along with .25 cc. of xylocaine without epinephrine. OT injectable is a liquid. It has a pH of around 2 to 4 and can cause significant burning pain when given, hence the use of the xylocaine. If within the first 2 to 3 minutes the patient feels his or her face becoming warmer and the ears warm, the patient would then seem to have adequate amounts of DHEA. The cells should respond to the use of oral OT tablets. It is still recommended that a DHEA sulfate level be drawn to get a baseline level on the patient. This will give a starting point for this particular patient's treatment.

During the first office visit a RBC magnesium level is drawn. If the RBC magnesium level is low, the patient should be started on Mag 200, two tablets twice daily. MAG 200 is a magnesium product that was developed to give the least amount of bowel irritation with excellent absorption.

Also measured at the first visit is the creatine blood level. If found low, replacement therapy is begun. Once the patient is responding to the therapy as listed in this paper, he or she can then be started on creatine monohydrate one teaspoon four times per day for one week, then two teaspoons every morning. Creatine can be mixed with juice, water, or applesauce. It is best given in the morning. If it is taken at night, it can keep an individual awake. Some patients with sensitive stomachs may have difficulty in taking creatine monohydrate and may need a lower starting dose.

If no blushing occurs at the time of giving the initial dose of oxytocin, patients are then requested to start on choline, inositol, and paba (five tablets per morning). Choline and inositol help load the enzymes that are being made by DHEA in order to help the inositol triphosphate system to respond to OT. Choline (1500 mg.) and inositol (1500 mg.) may also be found in the local health food stores.

At this point we need to focus on a new finding. As noted above, OT can stimulate the body to vasodilate its capillaries to give a person better circulation. Two recent medical papers have now shown that OT vasodilates the body's small blood vessels via the mechanism of stimulating production of nitric oxide. Nitric oxide is a very potent gas produced at the capillary level of the tissues. One of its major jobs is to improve tissue oxygenation. A few patients are having trouble making this gas, even in the presence of the hormones and nutrients thus far discussed.

During the last few months, we have learned to improve our therapy. We do this by giving sublingual nitroglycerin 1/2 tablet of .3 mg. every four hours. (Nitrostat .3 mg. sl q4hrs) This therapy can increase the blood supply to the brain, heart and tissues. A sign the therapy is working is when the patient develops a headache. This headache is due to increased blood supply to the brain. The headache will last one to fifteen minutes and then disappear. When the headache is gone, the individual will also notice a greater relief from their fibromyalgia pain. The pain relief will last about four to six hours before another sublingual tablet is required. The nitroglycerin works best in the presence of OT. If nitroglycerin is given by itself, a poor response may occur. The first pill should always be given in a doctor's office in case hypotension should develop. Therapy with nitroglycerin should always be started on those patients with weak or no blushing when given OT.

Since FMS patients have so much pain, they are placed on Super Malic, a malic acid and magnesium preparation that has undergone the rigors of a double-blind placebo-controlled trial and proven itself to be effective to reduce FMS pain. Three to six tablets twice per day is the recommended amount.[158] Currently in the USA there are many malic acid and magnesium preparations being sold. None of these have stood the rigors of medical testing to prove that they work. This is why only Super Malic can be recommended without reservation. The magnesium in Super Malic can encourage loose bowel movements, so it may be advisable to begin with one tablet three times a day, and eventually work up to a daily dose of three to four tablets three times a day, unless liquid stools develop. Increasing the dosage by one tablet per day every four to five days may be the best approach to use in the initial stages of treatment, when trying to establish an individualized dose response.

There seems to be a metabolic disturbance of the ability of the body to handle glucose in patients with FMS.[158] Because of this, patients are started on Super Malic to help correct the metabolism disorder in conjunction with DHEA.

Second Office Visit

After the patient has been on DHEA, magnesium, and Super Malic for three months and the inositol choline treatment, a challenge dose of intramuscular OT 10 U with lidocaine 1% 0.25 cc should be administered, unless the patient is sensitive to lidocaine or similar preparations. Within five minutes the patient should start to feel very warm and relaxed, and within twenty minutes notice a reduction of pain. Once the physician is satisfied that the patient has responded to OT, the patient can then start an oral dose of 10 U each morning. An upper limit of 40 U daily has been established for this therapy. Oral OT tablets were developed at Belmar Pharmacy from Lakewood, Colorado, and have been shown to be biologically active (unpublished data). Oral oxytocin tablets should be taken in the morning.

Observations at the office have also indicated that patients who smoke have not responded as well to the OT therapy. This is presumably because the chemicals in cigarette smoke may block OT receptors.

At the second office visit, repeat blood work should be done to monitor hormone and mineral blood levels for those patients that are receiving replacement therapy.

During the initial or subsequent office visits, many patients report a problem with a decreased desire for intimacy. This is a very private and understandably sensitive issue. However, we feel a responsibility to address the problem because so many women injured by FMS/CFIDS are affected; yet embarrassment and fear of further rejection prevent most from discussing it with treating physicians. It is important to realize that there are true physical reasons for this lack of desire, and that most women injured by FMS/CFIDS share this problem. Although medical opinions may differ as to the actual causes, the end results are essentially the same. No longer desiring to be intimate with a partner represents yet another insult from the ILLNESS, because it affects the well partner deeply, and it can affect the security of the marriage directly or indirectly.

Chronic illness imposes a real mix of limitations, experienced by both the injured and the well partner. It is as though personal identity and sense of purpose take up new residence in the background, as THE DISEASE and all that entails takes over. In addition, most families affected by FMS/CFIDS illness also suffer financial embarrassment, due either to mounting medical bills or to the sick partner's inability to work, or both. Adding the sick partner's chronically low or non-existent libido to this picture of intimacy for both partners is a challenge at best. However, striving to accomplish this can be absolutely devastating when perhaps the single most powerful ingredient for establishing and maintaining closeness has simply been removed.

For this reason, finding a treatment program with the potential to restore a healthy desire for intimacy, while at the same time reducing pain and increasing mobility, has seemed like an answered prayer to many chronically ill women.

Treatment Summary

Overall, FMS/CFIDS patients who are involved in this particular regimen seem pleased. However, as with any therapy involving medications, side effects do exist and should be researched before treatment is initiated. Although the information provided in this paper is accurate, it should by no means be considered complete.

Reported benefits of this therapy include a reduction of both pain and fatigue. Although still in the early stages, the above outlined interactive OT-Hormonal-Nutrient Treatment Protocol provides an exciting new alternative to the traditional methods of FMS/CFIDS treatment. Generally, mainstream medicine is geared toward treating symptoms. Because of time constraints, physicians may be more interested in reducing the severity of symptoms than identifying the cause. As identified earlier in the text, traditional methodology is now being challenged, as more and more FMS/CFIDS affected patients regain control over their lives and make a commitment to take an active role in their own recovery. As with anything else, it is important to conduct your own research, and decide on your own what seems to be the most reasonable approach for your personal treatment.

Side Effects

The following side effects have been associated in the medical literature with DHEA, Inositol, OT, Malic Acid, Magnesium:

DHEA/Side Effects

An increase in DHEA has been known to cause increased hair growth on the head, legs, underarms and the pubic area. (This is not normally considered to be a problem, because a decreased level of DHEA has usually created a reduction of hair growth in these areas.) This increase in hair growth can be witnesses by increased itching of the scalp and skin. The itching is actually secondary to the hair growth.

In addition, an increase of facial hair has been noted on rare occasions, but is not a frequently noted problem.

Because DHEA can also stimulate oil glands to increase oil production, an increase in acne may be seen.[159]

These side effects as listed are the natural effects of this hormone, so anytime an excess of DHEA is present, an increase in these areas can be expected.[68,70,98]

An increase in muscle mass and a slight increase in the fat mass around the abdomen has also been observed. (Clinical observation) If DHEA is taken at night, it can cause insomnia. This can be due to the fact that it is a neuroexcitatory hormone of the brain.[160-165]

Although DHEA is capable of increasing thermogenesis, patients receiving this hormone who normally complain of being hot all the time have reported feeling comfortably cooler. This would suggest that DHEA might play a role in helping to control the thermal settings of the brain which determine whether a patient is too hot or too cold.

DHEA/Undesirable Combination/Side Effects

The combination of thyroid hormone supplementation, DHEA, and injectable estrogen given to the same patient at the same time was noted to produce an overactive libido, to the extent the labia became painfully engorged. This extremely painful physical condition persisted for a period of 14 to 21 days. (clinical observation)

Oxytocin/Side Effects

OT therapy helps to stimulate the micro-circulation, thereby increasing body temperature which can make some patients feel uncomfortably warm.[10,54,166] Still, complaints of cold hands and feet are usually diminished, as the patient experiences increased circulation to these areas. Correct dose regulation can alleviate tissues that seem too warm.

OT therapy increases circulation to the head and can produce headaches, but they usually disappear within a short time after starting treatment.

Patients with congestive heart failure or decreased renal function are not good candidates for OT therapy because of its propensity to cause fluid retention.

OT should not be given to a pregnant patient as it may cause some fluid retention, or even miscarriage.

If a patient does not have enough DHEA or inositol on board at the time OT therapy is initiated, the addition of OT can actually cause agitation rather than produce its normal calming effect. This would suggest that this patient is not ready to begin OT therapy and would probably benefit from taking supplemental DHEA and inositol for a few months, before trying OT again.

On the other hand, too much OT could theoretically cause patients to experience a psychiatric problem known as obsessive compulsive disorder. This is based on data from one study only.[167]

In addition, an increase in the manic phase of patients diagnosed with manic-depressive illness is seen as a disorder of inositol.[125,127] This increase in the manic phase comes under quick control as soon as either the hormones or inositol are withdrawn.

Some patients have noted an increase in the size of breast tissue, sometimes necessitating a corresponding change in bra cup size. Increased breast and nipple tenderness have been reported by patients, while others report reduced breast tenderness before their monthly cycle. Patients have also reported greater sensation and sexual excitation when the breast is caressed.

Malic Acid/Magnesium/Side Effects

Gastric irritation can occur in the presence of malic acid.[158,168] Taking the nutrient with at least one eight ounce glass of water seems to minimize this reaction, although some still find it necessary to experiment until an appropriate personalized dosage of malic acid is reached.

Magnesium is contained in Super Malic and may cause problems with frequent loose bowel movements.[138,169] Many patients with constipation find this side effect of their therapy to be helpful. If liquid stools develop, reducing the Super Malic until two or three soft bowel movements per day are achieved seems to work well.

As previously described, this combination of preparations has been known to produce effects ranging from decreased fatigue and pain to clearer vision and improved thinking. Many symptoms are eliminated, such as being lightheaded, irritable bowel syndrome, cramps, cold hands and feet, foggy concentration, and muscle pain. Other improvements include better circulation, better temperature regulation, more energy, reduced skin sensitivity, and less agitation.

Please consider the above outlined plan for informational purposes only; patients are encouraged to use this as a starting point to further their own research for therapies which may bring them better health. If one is interested in this particular approach to treatment, this text with the above mentioned protocol can easily be taken to your own physician, who can initiate the program and monitor your progress.

As these and other treatment modalities surface, hope looms on the horizon for both women and men suffering from FMS/CFIDS related illnesses. The future holds even more promise!

Source of Medication

Belmar Pharmacy, Lakewood, Co., compounds a highly bioavailable form of DHEA as well as oxytocin. Both these hormones are available by prescription. Super Malic (Optimox Cooperation) is available without medical claims as a source of both malic acid and magnesium, and can be purchased at your local pharmacy or health food store as an over the counter product. It can also be purchased through Belmar, along with inositol/choline and Mag 200. The medication is shipped directly to the patient after a prescription has been faxed to the pharmacy from the doctor's office.

Orders should be faxed to: 303-763-9712

> Belmar Pharmacy
> 12860 W. Cedar Dr. #210
> Lakewood, Colorado 88228
> Telephone: 800-525-9473

Reprints of a publication featuring an open clinical trial with Super Malic can be obtained free of charge to your physician upon request from:

> Optimox Corporation
> P.O. Box 3378
> Torrance, California 90510-3378
> Telephone: 800-223-1601

Medication Orders *(should look like this)*

1. DHEA 50 mg. 1 qam #100 for DHEA levels less than 100mcg./dl.; 25 mg. of DHEA for levels between 100-200 mcg./dl.

2. Super Malic 3-6 bid #180.

3. Thyroid T3 60 or 90 mcg. 1 qam #100 (This pill is sustained release.)

4. Choline-Inositol-Paba 5 qam #250.

5. Mag 200 2 bid #120.

6. Oxytocin 10 unit tab 1-3 tab qam #100.

7. Creatine monohydrate 2 tsp. qam in juice #300 gms.; creatine should only be started after oxytocin has been initiated.

8. Nitrostat .3mg. sl q4-6hr #100; first dose should always be given in a doctor's office; try giving 1/2 tablet first.

Once the prescription is faxed to Belmar, have your patient call their 800 number to make financial arrangements to have the medications sent to them.

For more information about DHEA and Oxytocin therapy contact: Dr. Jorge D. Flechas, 724 5th Avenue West, Hendersonville, NC 28739; (704) 693-3015.

Your phone call will be returned as a collect call as time allows.

Special thanks is given to Sarah Templeton for her donated time and talent in originally typing this manuscript.

REFERENCES

1. Crofford, L.J., Pillemer, S.R., Kalogeras, K.T., Cash, J.M., Michelson, D., King, M.A., et al. Perturbations of Hypothalamic-Pituitary-Adrenal Axis Function in Patients with Fibromyalgia. *American College of Rheumatology*, 1993; 36:C195.

2. Crofford, L.J., Pillemer, S.R., Kalogeras, K.T., Cash, J.M., Michelson, D., Kling, M.A., et al. Hypothalamic-Pituitary-Adrenal Axis Pertubations in Patients with Fibromyalgia. *Arthritis & Rheum*, 1994; 37:1583-1592.

3. Demitrack, M.A., Dale, J.K., Straus, S.E., Laue, L., Listwak, S.J., Kruesi, J.P., et al. Evidence for Impaired Activation of the Hypothalamic-Pituitary-Adrenal Axis in Patients with Chronic Fatigue Syndrome. *Journal of Clinical Endocrinology and Metabolism,* 1991; 73:1224-1234.

4. Demitrack, M.A., Crofford, L.J. Hypothalamic-Pituitary-Adrenal Axis Dysregulation in Fibromyalgia and Chronic Fatigue Syndrome: An Overview and Hypothesis. *Journal of Musculoskeletal Pain,* 1995; 3:67-73.

5. Bakheit, A., Behan, P.O., Watson, W.S., Morton, J.J. Abnormal Arginine-Vasopressin Secretion and Water Metabolism in Patients with Postviral Fatigue Syndrome. *Acta Neurol Scand*, 1993; 87:234-238.

6. Crowley, W.R., Armstrong, W. Neurochemical Regulation of Oxytocin Secretion in Lactation. *Endocrine Reviews*, 1992; 13:33-65.

7. Amico, J.A., Robinson, A.G. The Radioimmunoassay of Oxytocin: New Developments. In: Amico, J.A,. Robinson, A.G., editors. *Oxytocin - Clinical and Laboratory Studies.* A.E. Amsterdam: Elsevier Science Publishers, B.V.. 1985:3-15.

8. Amico, J.A., Tenicela, R., Johnston, J., Robinson, A.G. A Time-Dependent Peak of Oxytocin Exists in Cerebrospinal Fluid but Not in Plasma of Humans. *Journal of Clinical Endocrinology and Metabolism,* 1983; 57:947-951.

9. Argiolas, A., Melis, M.R. Oxytocin-Induced Penile Erection: Role of Nitric Oxide. In: Ivell, R., Russell, J.A., editors. *OXYTOCIN: Cellular and Molecular Approaches in Medicine and Research.* New York: Plenum Press, 1995:247-254.

10. Suzuki, Y., Satoh, S.I., Kimura, M., Oyama, H., Asano, T., Shibuya, M., et al. Effects of Vasopressin and Oxytocin on Canine Cerebral Circulation in vivo. *J Neurosurg*, 1992; 77:424-431.

11. Oyama, H., Suzuki, Y., Satoh, S.I., Kajita, Y., Takayasu, M., Shibuya, M., et al. Role of Nitric Oxide in the Cerebral Vasodilatory Responses to Vasopressin and Oxytocin in Dogs. *Journal of Cerebral Blood Flow and Metabolism*, 1993; 13:285-290.

12. Katusic, Z.S., Shepherd, J.T., VanHoutte, P.M. Oxytocin Causes Endothelium-Dependent Relaxations of Canine Basilar Arteries by Activating V1-Vasopressinergic Receptors. *The Journal of Pharmacology and Experimental Therapeutics, 1985;* 236:166-170.

13. Mountz, J.M., Bradley, L.A., Modell, J.G. Fibromyalgia in women. Abnormalities of regional cerebral blood flow in the thalamus and the caudate are associated with low pain threshold levels. *Arthritis Rheum*, 1995; 38:926-938.

14. Henriksson, K.G. Aspects of the Pathogenesis of Chronic Muscular Pain. *Journal of Musculoskeletal Pain*, 1995; 3:35-41.

15. Hau, P.P., Scudds, R.A., Harth, M. An Evaluation of Mechanically Induced Neurogenic Flare by Infrared Thermography in Fibromyalgia. *Journal of Musculoskeletal Pain*, 1996; 4:3-20.

16. Moos, F,. Freund-Mercier, M.J., Guerne, Y., Stoeckel, M.E., Richard P. Release of oxytocin and vasopressin in Magnocellular Nuclei in Vitro: Specific Facilitatory Effect of Oxytocin on its Own Release. *Journal of Endocrinology*, 1983; 63:72.

17. Carmichael, M.S., Humbert, R., Dixen, J., Palmisano, G., Greenleaf, W., Davidson, J.M. Plasma Oxytocin Increases in the Human Sexual Response. *Journal of Clinical Endocrinology and Metabolism*, 1987; 64:27-31.

18. Pedersen, C.A., Caldwell, J.D., Jirikowski, G.F. Oxytocin and Reproductive Behaviors. In: Yoshida, S., Share, L., editors. *Recent Progress in Posterior Pituitary Hormones.* Amsterdam: Elsevier Science Publishers, B.V., 1988:141-149.

APPENDIX

19. Nussey, S.S., Page, S.R., Ang, V.T.Y., Jenkins, J.S. The Response of Plasma Oxytocin to Surgical Stress. *Clinical Endrocinology*, 1988; 28:277-282.

20. Altemus, M., Deuster, P.A., Galliven, E., Carter, C.S., Gold, P.W. Suppression of Hypothalmic-Pituitary-Adrenal Axis Responses to Stress in Lactating Women. *J of Clinical Endocrinology and Metabolism*, 1995; 2954-2959.

21. Gibbs, D.M. Vasopressin and Oxytocin: Hypothalamic Modulators of the Stress Response: A Review. *Psychoneuroendocrinology*, 1986; 11:131-139.

22. Burbach, P.H., Bohus, B., Gabor, L.K., Van Nispen, J.W., Greven, H.M., De Wied, D. Oxytocin Is A Precursor of Potent Behaviourally Active Neuropeptides. *European Journal of Pharmacology*, 1983; 94:125-131.

23. Clauw, D.J., Morris, S., Starbuck, V. Impairment in Cognitive Function in Individuals with Fibromyalgia. *Arthritis Rheum*, 1994; 37:s347

24. Kaplan, R.F., Meadows, M.E., Vincent, L.C. Memory impairment and depression in patients with Lyme encephalopathy. Comparison with fibromyalgia and nonpsychotically depressed patients. *Neurology*, 1992; 42:1263-1267.

25. Slotkoff, A.T., Clauw, D.J. Fibromylgia: When Thinking is Impaired. *The Journal of Musculoskeletal Medicine*, 1996; 32-36.

26. Yoshida, S., Share, L. Oxytocin and Experimental Drug Addiction: Receptor-Related Effects. In: Kovacs, G.L,. editor. *Recent Progress in Posterior Pituitary Hormones*, 1988. Amsterdam: Elsevier Science Publishers, B.V., 1988:127-132.

27. Gauquelin, G., Gharib, C., Krasnov, I.B., Geelen, G., Allevard, A.M., Brun, J., et al. Hypopyseal Hormones in the Retina, Pineal and Harderian Glands of the Rat. Modifications Induced by Environmental Factors. In: Yoshida S, Share L, editors. *Recent Progress in Posterior Pituitary Hormones*. Amsterdam: Elsevier Science Publishers, B.V, 1988:293-301.

28. Clauw, D.J. Fibromyalgia: More than just a Musculoskeletal Disease. *American Family Physician*, 1995; 52:843-851.

29. Rosenhall, U., Johansson, G., Orndahl, G. Eye Mobility Dysfunction in Chronic Primary Fibromyalgia with Dysesthesia. *Scand J Rehab Med*, 1987; 19:139-145.

30. Voloschin, L.M., Tramezzani, J.H. Milk Ejection Reflection Linked to Slow Wave Sleep in Nursing Rats. *Endocrinology*, 1979; 105:1202-1207.

31. Reiter, R.J., Robinson, J. Atypical Reactions. In: Reiter, R.J., Robinson, J, editors. *Melatonin: Your Body's Natural Wonder Drug*. New York: Bantam Books, 1995; 206-207.

32. Mayerhofer, A., Sterzik, K., Link, H., Wiemann, M., Gratzl, M. Effect of Oxytocin on Free Intracellular CA2+ Levels and Progesterone Release by Human Granulosa-Lutein Cells. *Journal of Clinical Endocrinology and Metabolism*, 1993; 77:1209-1214.

33. Behrens, O., Maschek, H., Kupsch, E., Fuchs, A.R. Oxytocin Receptors in Human Ovaries during the Menstrual Cycle. In: Ivell, R., Russell, J.A., editors. *OXYTOCIN: Cellular and Molecular Approaches in Medicine and Research*. New York: Plenum Press, 1995:485-486.

34. Legros, J.J., Chiodera, P., Geenen, V. Inhibitory Action of Exogenous Oxytocin on Plasma Coritsol in Normal Human Subjects; Evidence of Action at the Adrenal Level. *Neuroendocrinology*, 1988; 48:204-206.

35. Ang, V.T.Y., Jenkins, J.S. Neurohypophyseal Hormones in the Adrenal Medulla. *Journal of Clinical Endocrinology and Metabolism*, 1984; 58:688-691.

36. Hinson, J.P., Vinson, G.P., Porter, I.D., Whitehouse, B.J, Dept.of Biochemistry MC, Charterhouse Square, et al. Oxytocin and Arginine Vasopressin Stimulate Steroid Secretion by the Isolated Perfused Rat Adrenal Gland. *Neuropeptides*, 1987; 10:1-7.

37. Taylor, A.H., Whitley, G.S., Nussey, S.S. The Interaction of Arginine Vasopressin and Oxytocin with Bovine Adrenal Medulla. *Journal of Endocrinology*, 1987; 121:133-139.

38. Russell, I.J., Vipraio, G.A., Abraham, G.E. Serum Dehydroepiandrosterone Sulfate (DHEA) in Fibromyalgia Syndrome (FS) Rheumatoid Arthritis (RA), Osteoarthritis (OA) and Healthy Normal Controls (HC). *Arthritis & Rheumatism*, 1993; 36:S223.

39. Nilsson, E., de la Torre, B., Hedman, M. Blood DHEA-S levels in polymyalgia rheumatica/giant cell arteritis and primary fibromyalgia. *Clinical & Experimental Rheumatology*, 1994; 12:415-417.

40. Johnson, H., Torres, B. Regulation of Lymphokine Production by Arginine Vasopressin and Oxytocin: Modulation of Lymphocyte Function by Neurohypophyseal Hormones. *Journal of Immunology*, 1985; 135:773s-775s.

41. Johnson, H., Torres, B., Farrar, W. Vasopressin Replacement of Interleukin 2 Requirement in Gamma Interferon Production: Lymphokine Activity of a Neuroendocrine Hormone. *Journal of Immunology*, 1982; 139:983-986.

42. Geenen, V., Robert, F., Fatemi, M., Defresne, M.P., Boniver, J., Legros, J.J., et al. Vasopressin and Oxytocin: Thymic Signals and Receptors in T Cell Ontogeny. In: Yoshida, S., Share, L., editors. *Recent Progress in Posterior Pituitary Hormones*. Amsterdam: Elsevier Science Publishers, B.V., 1988:303-310.

43. Elands, J., Resink, A., De Kloet, E. R. Neurohypophyseal Hormone Receptors in the Rat Thymus, Spleen, and Lymphocytes. *Endocrinology*, 1990; 126:2703-2711.

44. Elands, J., Resink, A., De Kloet, E. R. Oxytocin Receptors in the Rat Thymic Gland. *European Journal of Pharmacology*, 1988; 151:345-346.

45. Geenen, V., Defresne, M.P., Robert, F., Legros, J.J,. Franchimont, P., Boniver, J. The Neurohormonal Thymic Microenvironment: Immunocytochemical Evidence that Thymic Nurse Cells Are Neurendocrine Cells. *Neuroendocrinology*, 1988; 47:365-368.

46. Caldwell, J.D., Walker, C., Noonan, L., Peterson, G., Pedersen, C.A., Mason, G. Thymic Oxytocin Receptors During Development and After Steroid Treatments in Adults. *Annals of the New York Academy Of Science*, 1995; 429-432.

47. Bussolati, G., Cassoni, P., Negro, F., Stella, A., Sapino, A. Effect of Oxytocin on Breast Carcinoma Cell Growth. In: Ivell, R., Russell, J.A. *CIN: Cellular and Molecular Approaches in Medicine and Research*. New York: Plenum Press, 1995:553-554.

48. Page, S.R., Ang, V.T.Y., Jackson, R., Nussey, S.S. The Effect of Oxytocin on the Plasma Glucagon Response to Insulin-

Induced Hypoglycemia in Man. *Diabetes & Metabolism,* 1990; 16:252.

49. Milenov, K., Kasakov, L. Effect of Synthetic Oxytocin on the Motor and Bioelectrical Activity of the Stomach and Small Intestines. *Acta Physiological Bulg,* 1979; 34:31-40.

50. Milenov, K. Effect of estradiol, progesterone and oxytocin on smooth muscle activity. In: Bulbring, E., Shuba, M.F., editors. *Physiology of Smooth Muscle.* New York: Raven Press, 1976:395-402.

51. McCarthy, M.M. Estrogen Modulation of Oxytocin and Its Relation to Behavior. In: Ivell, R., Russell, J.A., editors. *OXYTOCIN: Cellular and Molecular Approaches in Medicine and Research.* New York: Plenum Press, 1995:235-246.

52. Arletti, R., Bertolini, A. Oxytocin Acts as an Antidepressant in Two Animal Models of Depression. *Life Sciences,* 4195; 1725-1729.

53. Buchwald, D., Garrity, D. Comparison of patients with chronic fatigue syndrome: A comprehensive approach to its definition and study. *Arch Intern Med,* 1994; 154:2049-2053.

54. Argiolas, A., Gessa, G.L. Central Functions of Oxytocin. *Neuroscience & Biobehavioral Reviews,* 1991; 15:217-231.

55. Jenkins, J.S., Nussey, S.S. The Role of Oxytocin: Present Concepts. *Clinical Endocrinology,* 1991; 34:515-525.

56. Sukhof, R.R., Walker, L.C., Rance, N.E., Price, D.L., Young, III. Vasopressin and Oxytocin Gene Expression in the Human Hypothalamus. *J Comparative Neurology,* 1993; 337:306

57. Fabian, M., Forsling, M.L., Jones, J.J., Pryor, J.S. The Clearance and Antidiuretic Potency of Neurohypophyseal Hormones in Man and Their Plasma Binding and Stability. *J Physiol,* 1969; 204:653-668.

58. Pellegrino, M.J., Van Fossen, D., Gordon, C., Ryan, J.M., Waylonis, G.W. Prevalence of Mitral Valve Prolapse in Primary Fibromyalgia: A Pilot Investigation. *Arch Phys Med Rehabil,* 1989; 70:541-543.

59. Triadafilopoulos, G., Simms, R.W., Goldenberg, D.L. Bowel Dysfunction in Fibromyalgia Syndrome. *Digestive Diseases and Sciences,* 1991; 36:59-64.

60. Wilke, W.S. FIBROMYALGIA: Recognizing and addressing the multiple interrelated factors. *Postgraduate Medicine,* 1996; 100:153-170.

61. Hiltz, R.E., Gupta, P.K., Maher, K.A., Blank, C.A., Benjamin, S.B., Katz, P., et al. Low Threshold of Visceral Nociception and Significant Objective Upper Gastrointestinal Pathology in Patients with Fibromyalgia Syndrome. *Arthritis & Rheumatism,* 1993; 36:93.

62. Whitehead, W.E., Holtkotter, B., Enck, P., Hoelzl, R., Holmes, K.D., Anthony, J., et al. Tolerance for Rectosigmoid Distention in Irritable Bowel Syndrome. *Gastroenterology,* 1990; 98:1187-1192.

63. Granges, G., Littlejohn, G. Pressure Pain Threshold in Pain-Free Subjects, in Patients with Chronic Regional Pain Syndromes, and in Patients with Fibromyalgia Syndrome. *Arthritis and Rheumatism,* 1993; 36:642-646.

64. Lurie, M., Caidahl, K., Johansson, G., Bake B. Respiratory function in Chronic Primary Fibromyalgia. *Scand J Rehab Med,* 1990; 22:151-155.

65. Wallace, D.J. Genitourinary Manifestations of Fibrositis: An Increased Association with the Female Urethral Syndrome. *The Journal of Rheumatology,* 1990; 17:238-239.

66. Simm, R.W., Goldenberg, D.L. Symptoms Mimicking Neurologic Disorders in Fibromyalgia. *The Journal of Rheumatology,* 1988; 15:1271-1273.

67. Rainey, W.E., Bird, I.M., Mason, J.I., Carr, B.R. Angiotensin II Receptors on Human Fetal Adrenel Cells. *American Journal of Obstetrics and Gynecology,* 1988; 122:2012-2018.

68. Parker, L.N. Adrenarche and Puberty. In: Parker, L.N., editor. *Adrenal Androgens in Clinical Medicine.* San Diego: Academic Press, Inc., 1989:98-117.

69. Hornsby, P.J. Biosynthesis of DHEAS by the Human Adrenal Cortex and Its Age-Related Decline. In: Bellino, F.L., Daynes, R.A., Hornsby, P.J., Lavrin, D.H., Nestler, J.E., editors. *Dehydroepiandrosterone (DHEA) And Aging.* New York: Annals of the New York Academy of Sciences, 1995:29-46.

70. Parker, L.N. Skin Disease. In: Parker, L.N., editor. *Adrenal Androgens in Clinical Medicine.* San Diego: Academic Press, Inc. 1989:339-351.

71. Spector, T.D., Thompson, P.W., Perry, A., Grunnos, A.C. The Relationship Between Sex Steroids and Bone Mineral Content in Women Soon After Menopause. *Clin Endoc,* 1991; 34:37-41.

72. Szathmari, M. DHEA Hormone and Osteoporosis Prevention. *Osteoporosis Int,* 1994; 4:84-88.

73. Garg, M., Bondada, S. Reversal of age associated decline in immune response in PNU immune vaccine by supplementation with the steroid hormone DHEA. *Infect Immun,* 1993; 61:2238-2241.

74. Araneo, B.A,. Dowell, T., Diegel, M., Daynes, R.A. Dehydrotestosterone Exerts a Depressive Influence on the Production of Interleukin-4 and y-Interferon, But Not IL-2 by Activated Murine T Cells. *Blood,* 1991; 78:688-699.

75. Daynes, R.A., Araneo, B.A. Natural Regulators of T-Cell Lymphokine Production In Vivo. *Journal of Immunotherapy,* 1992; 12:174-179.

76. Ridson, G., Cope, J., Bennett, M. Mechanisms of Chemoprevention by Dietary Dehydroisoandrosterone. *American Journal of Pathology,* 1990; 136:759-769.

77. Ridson, G., Kumar, V., Bennett, M. Differential Effects of Dehydroepiandrosterone (DHEA) on Murine Lymphopoiesis and Myelopoiesis. *Exp Hematol,* 1991; 19:128-131.

78. Daynes, R.A., Dudley, D.J., Araneo, B.A. Regulation of Murine Lymphokine Production In Vitro. *Eur J Immunol,* 1990; 20:793-802.

79. Neifeld, J.P., Lippman, M.E., Tormey, D.C. Steroid Hormone Receptors in Normal Human Lymphocytes. *Journal of Biological Chemistry,* 1977; 252:2972-2977.

80. Parker, L.N., Levin, E.R., Lifrak, E.T. Evidence for Adrenocortical Adaptation to Severe Illness. *Journal of Clinical Endocrinology and Metabolism,* 1985; 947-952.

81. Gordon, G.B., Bush, T.L., Helzlsouer, K.J., Miller, S.R, Comstock, G.W. Relationship of Serum Levels of Dehydroepiandrosterone and Dehydroepiandrosterone Sulfate to the Risk of Developing Postmenopausal Breast Cancer. *Cancer Research,* 1990; 50:3859-3862.

82. Daynes, R.A., Araneo, B.A., Dowel, T.A. Regulation of Murine Lymphokine Production In Vivo. III The Lymphoid Microenvironment Exerts Regulatory Influences Over T Helper Function. *J Exp Med,* 1991; 171:979-996.

83. Gordon, G.B., Shantz, L.M., Talalay, P. Modulation of Growth, Differentiation and Carcinogenesis by Dehydroepiandrosterone. *Advances in Enzyme Regulation,* 1987; 26:355-383.

84. Henderson, E., Yang, J.Y., Schwartz, A. Dehydroepiandrosterone (DHEA) and Synthetic DHEA Analogs Are Modest Inhibitors of HIV-1 IIIB-Replication. *Aids Research and Human Retroviruses,* 1992; 8:625-631.

85. Jacobson, M.A., Fusaro, R.E., Galmarini, M., Lang, W. Decreased Serum Dehydroepiandrosterone Is Associated with an Increased Progression of Human Immunodeficiency Virus in Men with CD4 Cell Counts of 200-499. *Journal of Infectious Diseases,* 1991; 64:864-868.

86. Loria, R.M., Inge, T.H., Cook, S.S., Szakai, A.K., Regelson, W. Up-Regulation of the Immune Response and Resistance to Virus Infection with Dehydroepiandrosterone (DHEA). In: Lardy, H., Stratman, F., editors. *Hormones, Thermogenesis, and Obesity.* New York: Elsevier Science Publisher, B.V., 1989:427-437.

87. Schwartz, A.G., Whitcomb, J.M., Nyce, J.W., Lewbart, M.L., Pashko, L.L. Dehydroepiandrosterone and Structural Analogs: A New Class of Cancer Chemopreventive Agents. *Advances in Cancer Research,* 1988; 51:390-421.

88. Schwartz, A.G., Pashko, L.L., Whitcomb, J.M. Inhibition of Tumor Development by Dehydroepiandrosterone and Related Steroids. *Toxicologic Pathology,* 1986; 14:362.

89. Schwartz, A.G., Hard, G.C., Pashko, L.L., Abou-Gharbia, M., Swern, D. Dehydroepiandrosterone: An Anti-Obesity and Anti-Carcinogenic Agent. *Nutrition and Cancer,* 1981; 3:46-53.

90. Helzlsouer, K.J., Gordon, G.B., Alberg, A.J., Bush, T.L., Comstock, G.W. Relationship of Prediagnostic Serum Levels of Dehydroepiandrosterone and Dehydroepiandrosterone Sulfate to the Risk of Developing Premenopausal Breast Cancer. *Cancer Research,* 1992; 52:1-4.

91. Zumoff, B., Levin, J., Rosenfeld, R.S., Markham, M,. Strain, G.W., Fukushina, D.K. Abnormal 24-Hr. Mean Plasma Concentrations of Dehydroisoandrosterone and Dehydroisoandrosterone Sulfate in Women with Primary Operable Breast Cancer. *Cancer Research,* 1981; 41:3360-3363.

92. Stahl, F., Schnorr, D., Pilz, C., Dorner G. Dehydroepiandrosterone (DHEA) Levels in Patients with Prostatic Cancer, Heart Diseases and Surgery Stress. *Exp Clin Endocrinol,* 1992; 99:68-70.

93. Gordon, G.B., Helzlsover, K.J., Alberg. Serum levels of dehydroepiandrosterone and DHEA Sulfate and the risk of developing gastric cancer. *Cancer Epidemiol Biomakers Prev,* 1993; 2:33-35.

94. Gordon, G.B., Helzlsover, K.J., Comstock, G.W. Serum levels of DHEA and its sulfate, and the risk of developing bladder cancer. *Cancer Research,* 1991; 51:1366-1369.

95. Prough, R.A., Lei, X.D., Xiao, G.H., Wu, H.Q., Geoghegan, T.E., Webb, S.J. Regulation of Cytochromes P450 by DHEA and Its Anticarcinogenic Action. In: Bellino, F.L., Daynes, R.A., Hornsby, P.J., Lavrin, D.H., Nestler, J.E., editors. Dehydroepiandrosterone And Aging. *Annals of the New York Academy of Sciences,* 1995:187-199.

96. Milewich, L., Catalina, F., Bennett, M. Pieotropic Effects of Dietary DHEA. In: Bellino, FL, Daynes, R.A., Hornsby, P.J., Lavrin, D.H., Nestler, J.E., editors. Dehydroepiandrosterone And Aging. *Annals of the New York Academy of Sciences,* 1995:149-170.

97. Parker, L.N. Control of Adrenal Androgen Secretion. In: Parker, L.N., editor. *Adrenal Androgens in Clinical Medicine.* San Diego: Academic Press, Inc., 1989:30-57.

98. Parker, L.N., Odell, W.D. Control of Adrenal Androgen Secretion. *Endocrine Reviews,* 1980; 1:393-411.

99. McIntosh, M.K., Berdanier, C.D. Influence of Dehydroepiandrosterone (DHEA) on the Thyroid Hormone Status of BHE/cdb Rats. *J Nutr Biochem,* 1992; 3:194-199.

100. Schroick, E.D., Buffington, C.K., Hubert, G.D., Kurtz, B.R., Kitabchi, A.E., Buster, J.E., et al. Divergent Correlations of Circulating Dehydroepiandrosterone Sulfate and Testosterone with Insulin Levels and Insulin Receptor Binding. *Journal of Clinical Endocrinology and Metabolism,* 1988; 66:1329-1331.

101. Haning, Jr., R.V., Flood, C.A., Hackett, R.J., Loughlin, J.S., McClure, N., Longcope, C. Replacement of Dehydroepiandrosterone (DHEA) Enhances T-Lymphocyte Insulin Binding in Postmenopausal Women. *Fertil Steril,* 1995; 63:1027-1031.

102. Davis, S.R., Burger, H.G. Androgens and the Postmenopausal Woman. *J of Clinical Endocrinology and Metabolism,* 1996; 81:2759-2763.

103. Lardy, H., Su, C.Y., Kneer, N., Wielgus, S. Dehydroepiandrosterone Induces Enzymes that Permit Thermogenesis and Decrease Metabolic Efficiency. In: Lardy, H., Stratman, F., editors. *Hormones Thermogenesis and Obesity.* New York: Elsevier Science Publisher, 1989:415-426.

104. Song, M.K.H., Grieco, D., Rall, J.E., Nikodem, V.M. Thyroid Hormone Mediated Transcription Activation of the Rat Liver Malic Enzyme Gene by Dehydroepiandrosterone. *J Biol Chem,* 1989; 264:18985.

105. Marrarer, M,. Prough, R.A., Frenkel, R.A., Milewich, L. Dehydroepiandrosterone Feeding and Protein Phosphorylation, Phosphates, and Lipogenic Enzymes in Mouse Liver. *Proc Soc Exp Biol Med,* 1990; 193(2):110-117.

106. Sonka, J. *Acta Univ,* 1976; 71:146-171.

APPENDIX

107. Sonka, J., Stravkova, M. *Aggressologie 5, 1970*; 5:421-426.

108. Lanthier, A., Pantalioni, P. *J Steroid Biochem,* 1987; 28:697-701.

109. Dennenbaum, R., Hoffman, G., Oertel, G.W. *Horm Metab,* 1972; 4:383-385.

110. Hoffman, G., Modsches, B., Dohler, U. *Rach Derm Forsch,* 1972; 243:18-30.

111. Holzman, H., Krapp, R., Morsches, B. *Aerptliche Forsch,* 1971; 25:345-353.

112. Holzman, H., Morsches, B., Knapp, R., Hoffman, G. *Arch Derm Forsch,* 1973; 247:23-28.

113. Lang, R.E., Heil, W.E., Ganten, D., Hermann, K., Unger, T., Rascher, W. Oxytocin Unlike Vasopressin Is a Stress Hormone in the Rat. *Neuroendocrinology,* 1983; 37:314-316.

114. Koo, E., Feher, K.G., Feher, T., Fust, G. *Klin Woehenschr,* 1983; 61:701-717.

115. Felt, V., Starka, l. Metabolic Effects of Dehydroepiandrosterone and Atromid in Patients with Hyperlipaemia. *Corvasa,* 1966; 8:40-48.

116. Honer, W.G.T., Lightman, C. No Effect of Naloxone on Plasma Oxytocin in Normal Men. *Psychoneuroendocrinology,* 1986; 11:245-248.

117. Casson, P.R., Andersen, R.N., Herrod, H.G., Stentz, F.B., Straughn, A.B., Abraham, G.E., et al. Oral Dehydroepiandrosterone in Physiologic Doses Modulates Immune Function in Postmenopausal Women. *American Journal of Obstetrics and Gynecology,* 1994; 169:1536-1539.

118. Calabrese, V.P., Isaacs, E.R., Regelson, W. Dehydroepiandrosterone in Multiple Sclerosis: Positive Effects on the Fatigue Syndrome in a Non-Randomized Study. In: Kalimi, M., Regelson, W., editors. *Biologic Role of Dehydroepiandrosterone (DHEA).* New York: Walter de Gruyter, 1990:95-100.

119. Roberts, E., Fauble, T. Oral Dehydroepiandrosterone in Multiple Sclerosis: Results of a Phase One, Open Study. In: Kalimi, M., Regelson, W., editors. *Biologic Role of Dehydroepiandrosterone (DHEA).* New York: Walter de Gruyter, 1990:81-93.

120. Regelson, W., Kalimi, M., Loria, R.M. DHEA: Some Thoughts as to its Biologic and Clinical Action. In: Kalimi, M., Regelson, W., editors. *Biologic Role of Dehydroepiandrosterone.* New York: Walter de Gruyter, 1990:405-445.

121. Wolkowitz, O.M., Reus, V.I., Roberts, E., Manfredi, F., Chan, T., Ormiston, S., et al. Antidepressant and Cognition-Enhancing Effect of DHEA in Major Depression. In: Bellino, F.L., Daynes., R.A., Hornsby, P.J., Lavrin, D.H., Nestler, J.E., editors. *Dehydroepiandrosterone And Aging.* New York: Annals of the New York Academy of Science, 1995:337-339.

122. Russell, I.J., Michalek, J.E., Vipraio, G.A., Fletcher, E.M., Javors, M.A., Bowden, C.A. Serum Serotonin and Platelet 3H-Impramine Binding Receptor Density in Patients with Fibromyalgia/Fibrositis Syndrome. *J Rheum,* 1991.

123. Russell, I.J., Michalek, J.E., Vipraio, G.A. Serotonin [5HT] in Serum and Platelets [PLT] from Fibromyalgia Patients [FM] and Normal Controls. *Journal of Musculoskeletal Pain,* 1995; 3:144

124. Russell, I.J. Neurohormonal: Abnormal Laboratory Findings Related to Pain and Fatigue in Fibromyalgia. *Journal of Musculoskeletal Pain,* 1995; 3:59-65.

125. Fujii, E., Oku, M. Effects of Steroid Hormones on Change in [Ca2+] and on PI Response Following Oxytocin Stimulation in Cultured Human Myometrial Cells. *Acta Obst Gynaec Jpn,* 1995; 47:94-100.

126. Margolis, R.U., Press, R., Altszuler, N., Stewart, M.A. Inositol Production by the Brain in Normal and Alloxan-Diabetic Dogs. *Brain Research,* 1971; 28:535-539.

127. Berridge, M.J. Inositol Trisphosphate, Calcium Lithium and Cell Signaling. *JAMA,* 1989; 262:1834-1842.

128. Fein, A., Payne, R., Corson, D.W., Berridge, M.J., Irvine, R.F. Photoreceptor Excitation and Adaption by Inositol 1,4,5-Trisphosphate. *Nature,* 1984; 311:157-160.

129. Sakakibara, M., Alkon, D., Neary, J.T., Heldman, E. Inositol Trisphosphate Regulation of Photoreceptor. *MemJ Biophysial Society,* 1986; 50:797-803.

130. Ehrlich, B.E., Watras, J. Inositol 1,4,5 Trisphosphate Activates a Channel from Smooth Muscle Sarcoplasmic Reticulum. *Nature,* 1988; 336:583-586.

131. Irvine, R.F., Moor, R.M., Pollock, W.K., Smith, P.M., Wreggett, K.A. Inositol Phosphates: Proliferation, Metabolism and Function. *Phil Trans Soc Lond,* 1988; B320:281-298.

132. Berridge, M.J., Irvine, R.F. Inositol Trisphosphate: A Novel Second Messenger in Cellular Transduction. *Nature,* 1984; 312:315-321.

133. Busse, R., Mulsch, A., Fleming, I., Hecker, M. Mechanisms of Nitric Oxide Release from the Vascular Endothelium. *Circulation,* 1993; 87-V:18-25.

134. Goadsby, P.J., Kaube, H., Hoskin, K.L. Nitric Oxide synthesis couples cerebral blood flow and metabolism. *Brain Research,* 1992; 595:167-170.

135. Chowienczyk, P.J., Cockcroft, J.R., Ritter, J.M. Blood flow responses to intra-arterial acetylcholine in man: effects of basal flow and conduit vessel length. *Clinical Science,* 1994; 87:45-51.

136. Russell, I.J., Vipraio, G.A., Abraham, G.E. Red Cell Nucleotide [RCN] Abnormalities in Fibromyalgia Syndrome. *Arthritis and Rheumatism,* 1993; 36:S223.

137. Russell, I.J. Biochemical Abnormalities in Fibromyalgia Syndrome. *The Journal of Musculoskeletal Pain,* 1994; 2:101-115.

138. Abraham, G.E., Flechas, J.D. Management of Fibromyalgia: Rationale for the Use of Magnesium and Malic Acid. *Journal of Nutritional Medicine,* 1992; 3:49-59.

139. Clauw, D.J., Ward, K., Katz, P., Sunder, R. Muscle Intracellular Magnesium Levels Correlate with Pain Tolerance in Fibromyalgia (FM). *Arthritis and Rheumatism,* 1994; 37:R29.

140. Clauw, D., Blank, C., Hewett-Meulman, J., Katz, P. Low Tissue Levels of Magnesium in Fibromyalgia. *Arthritis and Rheumatism,* 1993; 61.

141. Bengtsson, A., Henriksson, K.G., Larsson, J. Reduced High-Energy Phosphate Levels in The Painful Muscles of Patients with

Primary Fibromyalgia. *Arthritis and Rheumatism*, 1986; 29:817-821.

142. Wortmann, R.L. Searching For The Cause of Fibromyalgia: Is There A Defect In Energy Metabolism? *Arthritis and Rheumatism*, 1994; 37:790-793.

143. McCully, K.K., Natelson, B.H., Iotti, S. J.S.J. Reduced Oxidative Muscle Metabolism in Chronic Fatigue Syndrome. *Muscle & Nerve*, 1996; May:621-625.

144. Bessman, S.P., Savabi, F. The Role of the Phosphocreatine Energy Shuttle in Exercise and Muscle Hypertrophy. In: Taylor, A.W., Golnick, P.D., Green, H.J., Ianuzzo, C.D., Noble, E.G., Metivier, G.S., editors. *Biochemistry of Exercise.* Champaign: Human Kinetics Publishers, 1990:167-178.

145. Spriet, L.L., Soderlund, K., Bergstrom, M., Hultman, E. Anaerobic Energy Release in Skeletal Muscle During Electrical Stimulation in Men. *American Physiological Society,* 1987; 611-615.

146. Wallimann, T., Wyss, M., Brdiczka, D., Nicolay, K. Intracellular Compartmentation, Structure and Function of Creatine Kinase Isoenzymes in Tissues with High and Fluctuating Energy Demands: The 'Phosphocreatine Circuit' for Cellular Energy Homeostasis. *Biochem J,* 1992; 281:21-40.

147. Boelen, A., Platvoet-ter, Shiphorst, M.C., Wiersinga, W.M. Soluble Cytokine Receptors and the Low 3,5,3' Triiodothyronine Syndrome in Patients with Nonthyroidal Disease. *J Clinical Endocrinology,* 1995; 80:971-976.

148. Szabolcs, I., Weber, M., Kovacs, Z., Irsy, G., Goth, M., Halzsz, T., et al. The Possible Reason For Serum 3,3'5' - (Reverse) Triiodothyronine Increase In Old People. *Acta,* 1982; 39:11-17.

149. Surks, M.L., Sievert, R. Drugs and Thyroid Function. *New England J Med,* 1995; 333:1688-1693.

150. Vagenakis, A.G. Division of Peripheral Thyroxine Metabolism From Activating To Inactivating Pathways During Complete Fasting. *J Clin Endocrine Metab,* 1975; 41:191-194.

151. Elliott, D.L. Sustained Depression of Resting Metabolic Rate After Massive Weight Loss. *Am J Clin Nutr,* 1989; 49 (1):93-96.

152. Komorowski, J. Increased Interleukin-2 Level in Patients with Primary Hypothyroidism. *Clinical Immunology & Immunopathology,* 1992; 63:200-202.

153. Arthur, J.R., Nicol, F., Beckett, G.J. Selenium Deficiency, Thyroid Hormone Metabolism, and Thyroid Hormone Deiodinases. *Am J Clin Nutr Suppl,* 1993; 57:236S-239S.

154. Wartofsky, L., Burman, K.D. Alterations in Thyroid Function in Patients with Systematic Illness: the "Euthyroid Sick Syndrome." *Endocrine Reviews,* 1982; 3:164-217.

155. Wilke, W.S., Sheeler, L.R., Makarowlki, W.S. Hypothyroidism Presenting Symptoms of Fibrositis. *Journal of Rheumatology,* 1987; 8:626-631.

156. Meeck, G., Riedel, W. Thyroid Function in Patients with the Fibromyalgia Syndrome. *Journal of Rheumatology,* 1992; 19:1120-1122.

157. Jurell, K.C., Zanetos, M.A., Orsinelli, A., Tallo, D., Waylonis, G.W. Fibromyalgia: A Study of Thyroid Function and Symptoms. *Journal of Musculoskeletal Pain,* 1996; 4:49-59.

158. Russell, I.J., Michalek, J.E., Flechas, J.D., Abraham, G.E. Treatment of Fibromyalgia Syndrome with Super Malic: A Randomized, Double Blind, Placebo Controlled, Crossover Pilot Study. *Journal of Rheumatology,* 1995; 22:5:953-958.

159. Qde, Raeve, L., De Schepper, J., Smitz, J. Prepubertal Acne: A Cutaneous Marker of Androgen Excess? *J of the American Academy of Dermatology,* 1995; 32:181-184.

160. Baulieu, E.E., Robel, P. Neurosteroids: A New Brain Function? *J Steroid Biochem Molec Biol,* 1990; 37:395-403.

161. Baulieu, E.E. Steroid Hormones in the Brain: Several Mechanisms. Fuxe, K., Gustafsson, J.A., Wetlerberg, L., eds. *Steroid Hormone Regulation of the Brain.* Oxford Pergamon, 1975; 3-14.1975; 3-14.

162. Robel, P., Baulieu, E.E. Neurosteroids Biosynthesis and Function. *Trends Endocrinol Metab,* 1994; 5:1-9.

163. McEwen, B.S. Steroid Hormones Are Multifunctional Messengers to the Brain. *Trends Endocrinol Metab,* 1991; 62-67.

164. Robel, P., Kawa, Y., Corpechot, C., Zhong-Yi, H., Jung-Testas, I., Kabbadj, K., et al. Neurosteroids: Biosynthesis and Function of Pregnenolone and Dehydroepiandrosterone in the Brain. In: Motta, M., editor. *Brain Endocrinology,* Second Edition. New York: Raven Press, Ltd., 1991:105-131.

165. Freiss, E., Trachsel, L., Guldner, J., Schier, T., Steiger, A., Holsboe, F. DHEA Administration Increases Rapid Eye Movement Sleep and EEG Power in the Sigma Frequency Range. *American Physiological Society,* 1995; E107-E13.

166. Altura, B.M., Altura, B.T. Vascular Smooth Muscle and Neurohypopyseal Hormones Oxytocin. *Federation Proceedings,* 1977; 36:1853-1860.

167. Leckman, J.F., Goodman, W.K., North, W.G., Chappell, P.B., Price, L.H., Pauls, D.L., et al. Elevated Cerebrospinal Fluid Levels of Oxytocin in Obsessive Compulsive Disorder. *Arch Gen Psychiatry,* 1994; 51:782-792.

168. Flechas, J.D. Clinical Effect of Super Malic (SM), a Malic Acid/Magnesium Oral Supplement, on Fibromyalgia Patients: Long Term Follow-up. *Journal of Musculoskeletal Pain,* 1995; 3:54.

169. Matz, R. Magnesium: Deficiencies and Therapeutic Uses. *Hospital Practice,* 1993; 79-92.

Medically reviewed and edited by Jorges D. Flechas, M.D., M.P.H.

Address: **Dr. Jorges D. Flechas**
724 5th Avenue West
Hendersonville, NC 28739
Phone (704) 693-3015 • Fax (704) 693-4471

APPENDIX

Effectively Treating
Severe Chronic Fatigue States

By Jacob Teitelbaum, M.D.

Dr. Teitelbaum is a leading clinician and researcher on effective treatment of CFIDS/FMS. His recent study, "Effective Treatment of Severe Chronic Fatigue States," showed that fibromyalgia is now a treatable disease! A larger, double-blind placebo-controlled study of his treatment protocol is scheduled to be completed in April 1998.

Dr. Teitelbaum is board certified in internal medicine. He practices and lives with his family in Annapolis, Maryland. His new book, From Fatigued to Fantastic – A Manual for Moving Beyond Chronic Fatigue and Fibromyalgia *and his newsletter are available by calling (800) 333-5287. He recently served as the state medical society appointee to the Maryland Governor's Commission on Complementary Medicine.*

An Overview

Chronic fatigue and immune dysfunction syndrome (CFIDS) and fibromyalgia syndrome (FMS) are two of many names for severe chronic fatigue states. These states overlap considerably and in most people result from a similar mix of processes.

My involvement with CFIDS/FMS began 20 years ago, when I came down with a severe viral syndrome while in medical school. I had always been an overachiever, with a "full-speed ahead" approach to life. A month into the illness, I was unable to even get out of bed before noon. Although my life had been dedicated to becoming a physician and healer, I was forced to withdraw from medical school.

With the help and support of my family and friends and the time to explore who I was, I recovered my energy and the strength to complete medical school and residency. Although doing well, I continued to intermittently have the many diverse symptoms seen in fibromyalgia. My experience with CFIDS and FMS left me with an appreciation of the impact of this illness. The symptoms that persisted (e.g., fatigue, achiness, poor sleep, bowel problems, etc.) acted as the arena in which I learned how to help people overcome the disease.

My father died of a massive heart attack at age 46. This left me with a strong interest in nutrition and preventive medicine. I also had a strong interest in endocrinology (hormone disorders). I've always loved massage. I learned the power of treating for myofascial (muscle) pain during my residency when a woman who had been in pain for over a decade was pain-free within seconds after I injected a distant trigger point. That incident motivated me to learn more about muscle disorders.

My patients have always been my best teachers. Their help, combined with an affinity for reading the scientific literature, has opened up many new areas to me. Over the years, my ability to help patients with CFIDS/FMS increased as more pieces of the puzzle fell into place. One day a patient brought in *The Trigger Point Manual.*[1] This text is the "bible" of muscle pain treatment. Chapter four of this two-volume book addresses "Perpetuating factors for myofascial pain." It turned out that this is what I had been treating.

If you have CFIDS, FMS or another disabling chronic fatigue state, you are on a difficult journey. I remember being told that I was depressed. I was—because I was unable to function. Most of us have struggled just to get compassion and understanding. Building on what I've learned by treating over 1,000 CFIDS/FMS patients since 1975, my research assistant Barbara Bird and I recently published a study of 64 patients with disabling chronic fatigue.[2] The majority had complete resolution of their fatigue with treatment, while most others had significant, albeit incomplete, improvement. Only four percent had no significant change. We found it took patients an average of less than seven weeks to start feeling better. Our current double-blind placebo-controlled study is scheduled to be completed in April 1998.

Our experience and research has shown that CFIDS/FMS patients have many underlying perpetuating factors. Five foundations of the illness are:

1. **Disordered sleep:** FMS is basically a sleep disorder associated with shortened, achy muscles with multiple tender knots. Trying to sleep on the tender knots is like trying to sleep on marbles. Because of this, people have trouble falling asleep and staying in the deep stages of sleep that recharge their batteries. Instead, they stay in light sleep and often wake up frequently during the night. Finally they fall fast asleep; five minutes later the alarm clock rings and they feel like killing it. If you have this problem, you may not have effectively slept for several years. When normal sleep is restored, people feel much better. I will note that sleeping pills (especially those in the Valium, Dalmane and Halcion family) actually worsen deep sleep. The day/night cycle is also disrupted in CFIDS/FMS. After being tired all day, people often find their mind is wide awake at bedtime.

2. **Hormonal disorders:** CFIDS and FMS are associated with fatigue via suppression of the hypothalamus gland. This is discussed at length in my book and first issue of my newsletter available from (800) 333-5287.[3,4] This suppression also occurs in viral infections. The hypothalamus is the body's master gland; it controls most of the other glands, including the adrenal, ovaries, testicles and thyroid glands. Suppression of the hypothalamus leads to a subtle, but disabling decrease in the function of many glands. People can even feel wiped out and have flu-like symptoms just from adrenal gland suppression. The hypothalamus also controls sleep, temperature regulation and autonomic function (causing low temperature and blood pressure).

For most people, suppression of the hypothalamus ends when the viral infection is over. Dr. William Jefferies theorized that people who remain chronically ill after a viral infection had long-term or permanent hypothalamus gland suppression.[5] He found that by treating these people with the adrenal hormone cortisol (in doses that are normal for the body), they often had marked improvement. Our research has supported this.

In most cases, hypothalamic suppression causes moderate suppression of several glands. Dr. Jefferies showed how this occurs. In his 1996 monograph, "Safe Uses of Cortisone,"[5] we see that the flu, for example, causes suppression of ACTH, the hormone which causes your adrenal gland to make adrenal hormone. Many fatigue symptoms are the result of adrenal suppression. When Dr. Jefferies gave fatigue and flu patients low doses of adrenal hormone, the flu-like symptoms often markedly improved.

Hormonal deficiencies can also occur in other ways. These include autoimmune disorders where the body mistakes parts of itself for an outside invader. A common triad occurs when the body attacks the thyroid and adrenal glands and the cells in the body that help you absorb Vitamin B_{12}.

Despite the glands being underactive, blood test results are often technically normal, albeit in the low range.[3,6] That is why many CFIDS/FMS patients have been told that their thyroid and adrenal glands are healthy, when indeed they are not. It is important to know how to interpret the tests and identify subclinical hormone deficiencies.

3. Immune dysfunction and recurrent infections: Although the immune system is not always suppressed in CFIDS or FMS, it usually is functioning poorly. My suspicion is that it is often on "overdrive" and then burns out. Although the cause of the immune dysfunction is not clear, there are many possibilities. Our experience suggests that although many infections (e.g., viruses, Lyme, mycoplasma, etc.) can trigger CFIDS, the immune and hormonal disorders persist even after the infection is gone. Recurrent respiratory and bladder infections and prostatitis are common. Bowel parasites (e.g., giardia, amoeba, cryptosporidium, etc.) are amazingly common. Frequent antibiotic treatments appear to cause not just vaginal but also bowel overgrowth of yeast, although this is a controversial area. These infections can cause the muscles to shorten and nutritional deficiencies to occur.

4. Nutritional deficiencies: These are potent triggers for fatigue, muscle shortening and immune dysfunction. Many CFIDS/FMS patients have found some symptomatic improvement just by taking nutritional supplements. B-vitamins (especially B_{12}), magnesium and iron deficiencies are especially important.

There are many causes for the nutritional deficiencies. These include:

A. Poor absorption: As noted above, this can come from overgrowth of yeast, parasites or unhealthy bacteria in the bowel which can absorb the vitamins and minerals before you can.

B. Overutilization: The body can overutilize nutrients when fighting infections in trying to repair damage from the illness.

C. Poor diet: We lose up to one-third of our vitamins and minerals (often more) to food processing. The average American has 140 pounds of sugar added to his/her diet each year. This accounts for 18% of calorie intake. White flour, which has been stripped of many micronutrients, accounts for another 18%. Less than five percent of Americans get the recommended daily intakes of copper, zinc and chromium, and the average American diet has less than one-half the magnesium of the average (unprocessed) Chinese diet. This is just the tip of the iceberg.

5. Mitochondrial dysfunction: Current evidence suggests that the mitochondria (the body's energy furnaces) are not working properly. This opens up many new exciting treatment

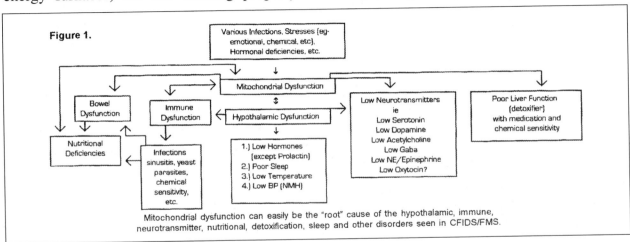

Figure 1.

Mitochondrial dysfunction can easily be the "root" cause of the hypothalamic, immune, neurotransmitter, nutritional, detoxification, sleep and other disorders seen in CFIDS/FMS.

possibilities. It may also be the common underlying cause of many of the above problems, plus other problems including low neurotransmitter (eg., serotonin, dopamine, etc.) levels.[7]

The Fatigue Cycle

Figure 1 shows the fatigue cycle. If you treat just one part, you may feel a bit better, but the overall problem persists. Our experience is that when you treat the whole cycle simultaneously, CFIDS/FMS resolves in over 50% of patients and significantly improves in about another 40%. For more information, see our study "Effective Treatment of Severe Chronic Fatigue States"[2] and abstract from the Myopain '95 Conference,[8] both published last year in *The Journal of Musculoskeletal Pain.*

So, How Do I Get Rid of It?

Most people are amazed at how quickly their symptoms improve (or resolve) when all their problems are treated simultaneously. The length and severity of the disease does not seem to affect recovery. To date, we have treated more than 1,000 patients over the last 15 years.

My new book, *From Fatigued to Fantastic – A Manual for Moving Beyond Chronic Fatigue and Fibromyalgia,*[3] details exactly which tests are needed, how to interpret them and how to treat CFIDS/FMS patients. My newsletter ($29.95/yr. from (800) 333-5287) has added many exciting, new treatment approaches. Following is a brief outline of my general CFIDS/FMS treatment protocol followed by a more in-depth treatment checklist. You will need to work closely with your primary care physician to determine what your personal protocol should be.

1. Stop sugar and caffeine intake. Six to nine months later, when you are consistently feeling well and any yeast overgrowth is resolved, you can have a modest amount of sweets. (No regular soda, though.) Many people seem to benefit from chocolate intake and don't always need to eliminate it. Decaffeinated coffee is okay if your bowels allow. Be prepared to go through withdrawal and feel awful the first week.

2. Limit alcohol. Some CFIDS patients cannot tolerate alcohol at all.

3. Take a good 25 mg. B-complex vitamin with minerals (such as those available through the CFIDS Buyer's Club, To Your Health and Natrol).

4. Magnesium/malic acid (I recommend Fibrocare from To Your Health). Take four to six tablets a day (less if diarrhea occurs). Take iron (not within six hours of any hormones) if your ferritin (iron) storage level is less than 40.

5. Sleep at least eight hours per night. Use low-dose Elavil, Flexeril, Ambien, Soma, Desyrel and/or (in severe cases because it is addictive) Klonopin as needed. Herbal remedies (including valerian 160-450 mg., melissa 80-160 mg., passiflora 80-180 mg., etc.) and melatonin .3 mg. are also helpful at bedtime. Unfortunately, herbal remedies alone are usually not strong enough for the severe sleep problems of CFIDS/FMS patients.

6. Slowly begin an exercise program as you improve. (Starting before treatment can cause next day "wipeout.")

7. Treat with Synthroid (25-75 mcg.) or Armour Thyroid (1/2-1 grain) each morning if symptoms suggest hypothyroidism (even if tests are normal).

8. Treat low or borderline adrenal function with Cortef and/or DHEA – even if the tests are low normal. Consider a trial of Florinef if blood pressure is low or the "tilt table test" is positive. (See the Fall '95 *Chronicle* – Editors.)

9. Consider treatment with estrogen in females or testosterone in males if these hormones are low. (See February '97 newsletter.[4])

10. Treat any bowel infections.

11. Treat any yeast overgrowth. Avoid antibiotics when possible.

12. Treat any sinusitis and/or nasal congestion. (Use the natural treatment discussed in my book.)

13. Consider vitamin B_{12} 2-3 mg. intramuscularly (I.M.) 1 to 3 times per week for 6 to 10 weeks, then as needed. I.V. nutritional treatments (Myers cocktails - I.V. magnesium, vitamin C, B-vitamins, etc.) can be dramatically beneficial.

14. For anxiety consider Desyrel.

15. For depression or frustration consider Paxil, Prozac or Zoloft. These may help even in the absence of depression. Begin with low doses. If these don't help or are poorly tolerated, try Wellbutrin.

16. Counseling is helpful to uncover life conflicts, etc. (I like Jungian.)

17. If fibromyalgia persists, consider sublingual nitroglycerin or Klonopin.

18. If fatigue persists, consider Coenzyme Q10, I.M. magnesium, or oxytocin plus treatment for mitochondrial dysfunction (see treatment checklist).

19. If problems persist, read Dr. Jay Goldstein's new book, *Betrayal by the Brain*, and try his protocol. Many other treatment options that can help in persistent cases are also reviewed in my *From Fatigued to Fantastic* book and newsletter[3,4,7] which contain the references for the data which provides the foundation for this approach.

In our experience, CFIDS and FMS are treatable illnesses. This includes resolution of the achiness, brain fog, bowel and sleep disorders and recurrent infections, as well as the fatigue. Increased thirst often persists (described as "drinking like a fish and peeing like a race horse!"). Although this could be treated with vasopressin, I prefer to just drink a lot of water and eat a lot of salt.

I think you will be amazed at what happens when you treat all of the underlying perpetuating factors simultaneously. Best wishes on becoming (or on watching your patients become) vibrant!

Dr. Teitelbaum's *From Fatigued to Fantastic* book ($11.95 + s&h) and newsletter ($29.95 for a three-issue year) are available from (800) 333-5287.

Treatment Protocol - CFIDS/Fibromyalgia

(Adapted from the book "From Fatigued to Fantastic" by Jacob Teitelbaum, M.D. - (800) 333-5287)

Dear patient,

Below is a listing of the more common treatments used in treating CFIDS/FMS. Although it can take 6 weeks to see a treatment's benefits, any side effects will often occur within the first few days of starting a treatment. Add in one new treatment each 1 to 3 days. If a side effect occurs, stop the last 2 or 3 treatments for a few days and see if it goes away. If the side effect is worrisome, call us or your family doctor (or go to the E.R.) immediately. If needed, all treatment can be stopped until the situation is clarified. Do not get pregnant on treatment or drive if sedated.

Nutritional Treatments

___ 1. Natrol's "My Favorite Multiple-Take One" (has to have those exact 5 words on the label), 1 a day.

___ 2. Fibrocare (magnesium/malic acid), 2 tablets 3 x a day for 8 months, then 2 tablets a day (less if diarrhea is a problem). From "To Your Health" company, (800) 801-1406.

___ 3. Calcium, 500 to 1000 mg. daily with 400 units of vitamin D (a chewable calcium or Oscal or Caltrate is recommended). Take if on Cortef.

___ 4. Chromagen (iron) one tablet a day. Do not take within 6 hours of any hormone preparations, as this can prevent their absorption. Take on an empty stomach. It is OK to miss up to 3 doses a week. Stop in 4 to 6 months.

___ 5. Vitamin B_{12}, 1 shot (2000 mcg.) ___ times weekly for___weeks, then as needed or ____ mcg. under your tongue daily.

Mitochondrial Energy Treatments – Use these for 10 to 12 weeks. Then drop the dose to the lowest dose that maintains the effect (or stop it if no benefit).

___ 1. Acetyl-L-carnitine, 1000 mg.- 2 x a day for 3 months. Then 250 to 500 mg./day or stop it.

___ 2. Coenzyme Q10, 100 to 200 mg. - 1 x a day.

___ 3. L-Lysine, 1000 mg. - 3 x a day for 3 months, then 1000 mg. a day.

___ 4. Magnesium/potassium aspartate, 2 capsules - 2 x a day (need to use a "fully reacted" brand).

___ 5. NADH (use Enada brand), 5 mg. - 2 tablets each morning. Take it on an empty stomach first thing in the morning at least 1/2 hour before eating or taking any medication or supplements.

___ 6. My-B-Tabs (ATP), 50 mg. - dissolve under your tongue 3 x a day.

___ 7. Thiamine pyrophosphate (cocarboxylase), 100 mg. shot (I.M.) 3 x a week for ____ weeks.

___ 8. Creatine Monohydrate, 5 gm. (5000 mg.) - 4 x a day for 5 days, then either ____ repeat the above first five days of each month or ____ take 2 gm. a day.

APPENDIX

___ 9. B-complex, 50 mg. - ____ tablet(s) at night.

___ 10. NAC (N-acetyl-cysteine) 500 mg. a day and/or glutathione 250 mg. a day.

Sleeping Aids for Fibromyalgia – Adjust dose as needed to get 7 to 8 hours of solid sleep without waking or hangover. No going to the bathroom if you wake up unless you still have to go 10 minutes later. Mixing low doses of several treatments is more likely to help you sleep without a hangover than a high dose of one medication. You can take up to the maximum dose of all checked off treatments simultaneously. Do not drive if you have next day sedation. If you're not sleeping 7 to 8 hours a night without waking on the checked off treatments, do **not** wait until your next appointment to let us know!

___ 1. Elavil (amitriptyline) 10 mg. - 1/2 to 5 tablets at bedtime.

___ 2. Flexeril (cyclobenzaprine) 10 mg. - 1/2 to 2 at bedtime.

___ 3. Desyrel (trazodone) 50 mg. - 1/2 to 6 at bedtime.

___ 4. Ambien, 10 mg. - 1/2 to 1 at bedtime.

___ 5. Benadryl (diphenhydramine) 25 to 50 mg. at night.

___ 6. Xanax, 1/2 mg. - 1/2 to 4 tablets at bedtime.

___ 7. Melissa (lemon balm), 80 to 160 mg. plus Valerian 180 to 360 mg. (available from "To Your Health" as "Valerian Rest").

___ 8. Melatonin, .3 mg. - 1 at bedtime (available at health food stores).

___ 9. Klonopin (clonazepam), 1/2 mg. - begin slowly and work your way up as sedation allows, 1/2 tablet at bedtime increasing up to 4 tablets at bedtime as needed.

___10. Soma (carisprodol), 1/2 to 1 at bedtime.

Hormonal Treatments

___ 1. Synthroid, ____ mcg. - one each morning (do not take within 6 hours of an iron supplement, except for the iron in your multivitamin). Begin with 1/2 tablet each morning the first week. (See #2 below.)

___ 2. Armour Thyroid, ____ grain - ____ tablets each morning. Begin with 1/4 grain a day for the first week and 1/2 a grain a day for the next 4 weeks; then you can go as high as 1 grain a day. Adjust it to the dose that feels best and recheck thyroid blood tests after 6 weeks on this dose. If caffeine-like shakiness occurs, lower the dose. If chest pain or increased palpitations occur, stop the thyroid and call us or your family doctor (or go to the E.R.) immediately.

___ 3. Cortef, 5 mg. tablets - ____ tablet(s) at breakfast, ____ at lunch, ____ at 4 P.M.

___ 4. DHEA, ____ mg. each morning (lower the dose if acne or darkening of facial hair occurs).

___ 5. Florinef, 0.1 mg. - 1 each morning. Begin with 1/4 tablet and increase by 1/4 tablet each 3 to 7 days.

Increase more slowly if headache occurs. Increase your water, salt and potassium (e.g., 12 oz. V-8 juice and one banana a day) intake.

___ 6.   Oxytocin, 10 units each morning.

___ 7.   Natural estrogen, ____ take Estrace (estradiol) ____ mg. ____ times a day, **OR**____ put a Climara ____ mg. patch on each Sunday, **OR** take a Triestrogen ____ mg. ____ times a day.

___ 8.   Ortho-novum 1/35 - begin the Sunday after this period.

___ 9.   Natural Progesterone, 100 mg. daily **OR** 200 mg. a day for the 16th to 25th day of your cycle. (Take at bedtime)

___10.   Testosterone, ____ mg. a day by mouth **OR** ____ mg. (____ cc) shot every ____ days.

Antiviral Agents

___ 1.   Valtrex, 500 mg. - 3 x a day. If you are feeling better in 1 month, continue Valtrex until you feel well for 2 more months. If you're not better in 1 month, stop it.

___ 2.   Echinacea, 300 to 325 mg. - 3 x a day while on Valtrex. Stay off the echinacea 1 week each month (or it will stop working).

___ 3.   Monolaurin, 300 mg. capsules. Take 9 capsules once a day on an empty stomach for 1 week, followed by 6 capsules once a day for 20 days. Take Lysine 1500 mg. twice a day while on Monolaurin.

Anti-Yeast Treatments

___ 1.   Avoid sweets - this includes sucrose, glucose, fructose, corn syrup, or any other sweets until the doctor says that it is okay to include them in your diet again. Avoid fruit <u>juices</u>, which are naturally sweet. Having 1 to 2 fruits a day (the whole fruit as opposed to the juice) is okay. Stevia is wonderful (it is an herbal sweetener - available from (800) 478-3842) – use all you want.

___ 2.   Acidophilus or other milk bacteria. Four billion units a day (refrigerated). Do **<u>not</u>** take while taking antibiotics.

___ 3.   Nystatin, 500,000 units - 2 tablets 3 x a day. Begin with 1 a day and increase by 1 tablet a day until you are up to the total dose. Your symptoms may initially flare as the yeast die off. If this occurs, increase the Nystatin more slowly or stop for a while until symptoms decrease. The Nystatin is usually taken for 5 months.

___ 4.   Sporanox, 100 mg. - begin taking this 4 weeks after beginning the Nystatin. Take 2 each day (simultaneously) with food for 6 weeks. If the symptoms have improved and then worsen when you stop the Sporanox, refill the prescription for another 6 weeks. (Note: A 6-week supply costs over $500!) If your symptoms flared when you began the Nystatin, begin with 1/2 to 1 capsule a day for the first week. **Do not take Seldane, Hismanyl, Propulcid or antacids (e.g., Tagamet) while on Sporanox!** Diflucan may be substituted for Sporanox if you are on antacids.

Treatment for Parasites and Other Infections

___ 1. Flagyl (metronidazole), ____ mg. 3 x a day for ____ days. Do not drink alcohol while on this medication as it will make you vomit.

___ 2. Yodoxin, 650 mg. - 3 x a day for 20 days after Flagyl is completed.

___ 3. Artemesia annua (an herbal antiparasitic), 500 mg. - 2 tablets 3 x a day for 20 days.

___ 4. Tricyclin (an herbal antiparasitic), 2 tablets 3 x a day after meals for 6 to 8 weeks.

___ 5. Colostrum (mother's milk), 3 capsules 3 x a day for 8 to 12 weeks, then stop or use the lowest dose needed for symptoms. If nausea or indigestion occurs, lower the dose to a comfortable level for 1 to 2 weeks until it passes. Take on an empty stomach.

___ 6. Doxycycline, 100 mg. - 2 x a day for 6 weeks. If symptoms <u>recur</u> when the Doxycycline is completed, keep repeating 6-week courses until the symptoms stay resolved. Take Nystatin (at least 2 twice a day) while on the antibiotic.

Nonspecific Treatments

___ 1. Nitroglycerin, 1/4 to 1 tablet dissolved under the tongue as needed for muscle pain.

___ 2. Rhus tox (homeopathic treatment), dissolve under the tongue as directed on the bottle as needed for muscle pain.

___ 3. Zoloft, ____ mg. - ____ tablet(s) each morning or evening.

___ 4. Paxil, 20 mg. ____ tablet(s) each morning.

___ 5. Prozac, 20 mg. - ____ tablet(s) each morning.

___ 6. Effexor, 37½ mg. - ____ times a day.

___ 7. Serzone, 100 mg. - 2 x a day for 1 week, then 150 mg. 2 x a day.

___ 8. Wellbutrin, ____ mg. - ____ x a day.

___ 9. MSM (sulfur=methyl sulfonyl methane), 1000 mg. - 3 tablets 2 x a day for 2 to 3 months, then as needed.

___ 10. Hypericum (St. John's Wort), 300 to 325 mg. - 3 x a day (takes 6 weeks to see effect - also works as an antidepressant).

___ 11. Parlodel (Bromocriptine), 2½ mg. - 1/2 tablet at night for first week, then 1 tablet at night.

___ 12. Baclofen, ____ mg. ____ times a day.

Follow-Up Testing

___ 1. Stool O&P or _____ in ____ week(s).

___ 2. Sleep apnea study.

___ 3. DHEA - Sulphate level in ____ weeks.

___ 4. Free T4, total T3, TSH levels in ____ weeks.

___ 5. Potassium level in ____ weeks.

___ 6. Free testosterone level in ____ weeks.

___ 7. Prolactin level in ____ weeks.

REFERENCES

1. Travell, J.G., Simons, D.G. *The Trigger Point Manual.* Williams & Wilkins, 1983.
2. Teitelbaum, J., Bird, B. Effective treatment of severe chronic fatigue: a report of a series of 64 patients. *J Musculoskel Pain,* 1995; 3(4), 91-110.
3. Teitelbaum, J. *From Fatigued to Fantastic.* Avery Press, 1996. (See item 3220 on page 63-64).
4. Teitelbaum, J. *From Fatigued to Fantastic.* Newsletter, February 1997.
5. Jefferies, W. *Safe Uses of Cortisol.* Charles C. Thomas Publishing, 1996.
6. Neeck, G., Riedell, W. Thyroid function in patients with fibromyalgia syndrome. *J Rheum,* 1992; 19:1120-22.
7. Teitelbaum, J. *From Fatigued to Fantastic.* Newsletter, July 1997.
8. Teitelbaum, J. Effective treatment of severe chronic fatigue states. *J Musculoskel Pain,* 1995; 3(1):28.

Medically reviewed and edited by Jacob Teitelbaum. M.D.

Address: **Dr. Jacob Teitelbaum**
466 Forelands Road
Annapolis, MD 21401
Phone: (410) 573-5389 • Fax (410) 266-6104
website: http://www.endfatigue.com

A Typical Neurosomatic New Patient Treatment Protocol

By Jay Goldstein, M.D.

Jay Goldstein, M.D., is director of the Chronic Fatigue Syndrome Institute in Anaheim, California. He has treated many CFIDS/FMS patients and has authored a variety of works on these conditions. He is the author of Chronic Fatigue Syndromes: The Limbic Hypothesis *and* Betrayal by the Brain: The Neurologic Basis of Chronic Fatigue Syndrome, Fibromyalgia Syndrome, and Related Neural Network Disorders.

AGENTS TRIED SEQUENTIALLY	ONSET OF ACTION	DURATION OF ACTION
1. Naphazoline HCI 0.1% gtt - OU	2 - 3 seconds	3 - 6 hours
2. Nitroglycerine 0.04 mg. sublingual	2 - 3 minutes	3 - 6 hours
3. Nimodipine 30 mg. po	20 - 40 minutes	4 - 8 hours
4. Gabapentin 100 - 800 mg. po	30 minutes	5 - 9 hours
5. Baclofen 10 mg.	30 minutes	8 hours
6. Topiramate 25 - 50 mg.	45 minutes	12 - 24 hours
7. Tiagabine 4 mg.	30 minutes	12 - 24 hours
8. Hydergine 2 mg.	30 minutes	8 hours
9. Tramadol 50 - 100 mg.	30 minutes	4 - 6 hours
10. Oxytocin 5 - 10 U IM QD or BID	15 minutes - 72 hours	12 - 24 hours
11. Pyridostigmine 30 - 60 mg. po	30 minutes	4 - 6 hours
12. Hydralazine 10 - 25 mg. po	30 - 60 minutes	6 - 12 hours
13. Mexiletine 150 mg. po	30 - 45 minutes	6 - 8 hours
14. Tacrine 10 - 20 mg. plus Donepezil 5 mg. HS po	30 minutes	4 - 6 hours
15. Risperidone 0.25 - 0.5 mg.	45 - 60 minutes	12 - 24 hours
16. Pindolol 5 mg.	15 - 30 minutes	12 hours
17. Lamotrigine 25 - 50 mg.	30 - 45 minutes	24 hours
18. Papaverine SA 150 - 300 mg. BID po	30 minutes - 4 weeks	12 hours
19. Sumatriptan 3 - 6 mg. SQ or 50 mg. po or 20 mg nasally	15 - 30 minutes	16 hours
20. Ranitidine 150 mg.	1 hour - 1 week	12 - 24 hours
21. Phentermine 8 mg.	30 minutes	8 hours
22. Olanzapine 2.5 - 10 mg.	45 minutes	24 hours
23. Cycloserine 15 - 50 mg.	15 - 30 minutes	24 hours
24. Tizanidine 2 - 4 mg.	20 - 30 minutes	4 hours
25. Felbamate 400 mg	30 minutes	6-8 hours
26. Lidocaine 240 - 480 mg. in 500 ml. normal saline infused over 2-3 hours	Immediate - 48 hours	2 hours - 2 weeks
27. Ketamine 25 mg. in 500 ml. normal saline infused over 2-3 hours	Immediate-48 hours	2 hours - 2 weeks
28. Thyrotropin releasing hormone 500 units in 9 ml. normal saline by slow I.V. push	Immediate	1 day - 3 weeks
29. Honey bee venom 25 - 50 mcg SQ	10 minutes	1 day - 1 week
30. Ascorbic acid 25 - 50 Gm + Ca gluconate 1 Gm + $MgSo_4$ 1 Gm in 400 ml normal saline infused over 2 -3 hours	Immediate - 1 day	1 day - 1 week

I halt sequential trials when the patient is virtually asymptomatic, using other medications if tolerance should develop. These drugs are all relatively free of adverse reactions and do not appreciably interact with one another. A patient taking tacrine requires regular liver function tests. Because of reports of aplastic anemia, felbamate therapy should be monitored with bi-weekly blood counts and liver function tests. The total daily dose of gabapentin may be as high as 5,000 mg. if lower doses are not beneficial. Using this protocol, most patients are dramatically improved in one or two office visits.

DISCLAIMER: Medicine is an ever-changing science. As new research and clinical experience broaden our knowledge, changes in treatment and drug therapy are required. While many suggestions for drug usage are made herein, this article is intended for educational purposes only, and the author, editor and publisher do not accept liability in the event of negative consequences incurred as a result of information presented in this article. We do not claim that this information is necessarily accurate by the rigid, scientific standard applied for medical proof, and therefore make no warranty, express or implied, with respect to the material herein contained. Therefore the patient is urged to consult his or her own physician prior to following a course of treatment. The physician is urged to check the product information sheet included in the package of each drug he or she plans to administer to be certain the protocol followed is not in conflict with the manufacturer's insert. When a discrepancy arises between these inserts and information in this article, the physician is encouraged to use his or her best professional judgment.

APPENDIX

Medically reviewed and edited by Jay A. Goldstein, M.D.

Address: **Dr. Jay A. Goldstein**
701 North Glassell Street
Orange, California 92867
Phone: (714) 516-2830 • Fax (714) 516-2707

Protocol for Fibromyalgia Treatment

By Thomas J. Romano, M.D., Ph.D., FACP, FACR

Dr. Romano is a compassionate and dedicated rheumatologist living and practicing in Wheeling, West Virgina. He has treated many FMS patients, authored a number of research articles on the topic and is very interested in the treatment of fibromyalgia. He serves on the Board of Advisors of the American Academy of Pain Management and is on the editorial board of the Journal of Musculoskeletal Pain.

My approach to the fibromyalgia (FMS) patient is very similar to that of Travell and Simons with regard to patients with myofascial pain. That is, perpetuating factors need to be identified and eliminated/ameliorated in order for the patients to benefit from medical intervention. Typically, I look for nutritional inadequacies, metabolic and endocrine inadequacies, psychological factors, postural problems, concomitant inflammatory diseases such as lupus or rheumatoid arthritis, etc. and should one or several of these problems exist, all efforts should be made to correct the situation in order for the FMS treatment to be successful. For example, some patients with FMS have vitamin deficiencies typically of one or more of the B vitamins or vitamin C or they have an excessive amount of vitamin A.   Some FMS patients have extremely poor posture while others may have low levels of Dehydroepiandrosterone (DHEA), growth hormone, thyroid hormone or have other types of hormone imbalances. Of course, a FMS patient may have none, a few or many of these possible perpetuating factors, so a careful history and physical examination should be done and appropriate testing be performed. Naturally, not every FMS patient can be tested for every conceivable perpetuating factor, but some elements of the history can tip off a clinician and point to a reasonable course of investigation.   For example, a patient taking diuretics on a chronic basis might develop hypomagnesemia, hypokalemia or other electrolyte imbalances. A patient who complains of being cold might have low serum ferritin or a low level of thyroid hormone. A thorough history and physical examination are critical and can alert the clinician to possible perpetuating factors. In a patient whose FMS seems to be resistant to medical intervention getting vitamin levels is a reasonable strategy. I have observed that many patients with vitamin imbalances respond better to medical treatment after their vitamin imbalances are corrected.

Once perpetuating factors have been dealt with, I aim at correcting the stage four non-REM delta wave sleep disorder that seems to be characteristic of the vast majority of, if not all, FMS patients. Medications such as tricyclic drugs, serotonin reuptake inhibitors, mild tranquilizers, can all be used effectively in helping to alleviate the sleep disorder. I tend to question the patient about "jerking" at bedtime. This can alert the clinician that the patient may have nocturnal myoclonus and that the patient's abnormal movements may actually be interfering with stage four sleep. If the patient gives such a history or if the patient's spouse notices that the patient "jerks" or "twitches" at night, then a trial of Klonopin 0.5 mg. po qhs will be a reasonable way of suppressing these abnormal movements, thus allowing the patient to sleep more normally. I frequently use medications for pain. I tend to use the nonacetylated salicylates such as Trilisate® or Disalcid® at a dose of up to 3 grams per day.   These are anti-inflammatory medications with analgesic properties. They are selective prostaglandin inhibitors so they do not predispose the patient to peptic ulcer disease, renal plasma flow problems (which could cause difficulty with fluid retention) and they do not thin the blood or cause easy bruising. Therefore they are the safest of all anti-inflammatories and seem to be fairly effective if used in conjunction with other medications for the treatment of patients with FMS. Newer pain medications such as Tramadol

(Ultram®) can also be useful if given in doses of approximately 50 mg. every four to six hours as needed for pain. I encourage the use of aerobic exercise where appropriate. Some patients are so deconditioned that they cannot do aerobics on land but need to start with an aquacise or water aerobics program and then graduate to more vigorous activity, but this should be done gradually and slowly so as not to cause relapses. One must, of course, understand that weather changes, increased activity, emotional stress, etc., can all make symptoms of FMS worse, so these must be taken into account in designing any type of exercise program. Furthermore, patients with myofascial bands, trigger points and muscle spasm may be unable to exercise on certain days or perform certain activities so the patient must be thoroughly examined for these and these should be dealt with accordingly. I tend to use tender point and/or trigger point injections in my practice as the situation dictates. I don't think there is any ironclad rule one way or the other regarding the use of these injections, but I let the patient's condition dictate the type of therapy. For example, some FMS patients have no trigger points and their muscles do not appear to be very tight most of the time. These patients probably would not benefit from soft tissue injections. However, there are many fibromyalgia patients that have concomitant myofascial pain syndromes with trigger points, myofascial bands and spasm. Injection of such trigger points can be very useful in alleviating specific niduses of musculoskeletal pain.

I instruct my patients to obtain a book called *Pain Erasure* by Bonnie Prudden, Ballantine Books, New York, 1980. This book is a very useful manual in that it teaches patients why muscles get tight, how massage and myotherapy (i.e., ischemic compression) can be helpful and can serve as a good handbook for deep tissue massage. Oftentimes a member of the household, such as the patient's spouse or friend, can perform this treatment with good temporary relief of pain. I also use a lotion called Aurum® lotion. It has been shown to be of help in patients with FMS and applying this lotion and massaging it into painful tight muscles three to four times a day has helped to ease pain in many of my patients. However, there are some patients that require the use of professional massage therapists to help ease muscle pain. I certainly would encourage this. However, I rarely ask the patients to see a massage therapist with no follow-up at home. Rather, I encourage the patient to use a massage therapist as a resource in getting rid of the most recalcitrant areas of muscle spasm and tightness, whereas most of the areas of tight muscle can be treated at home with regular massage and stretching.

I encourage FMS patients to ask questions, especially about new modalities, nutritional supplements, etc. However, I stress to the patient that one particular medication or mode of therapy is often insufficient in controlling most of the symptoms. Rather, a combination of avoidance of perpetuating/aggravating factors, the enhancement of stage four sleep, the use of anti-inflammatories/analgesic medication and/or the use of muscle relaxants, the "hands-on" treatment, such as myotherapy/ischemic compression and massage therapy, as well as the judicious use of injections need to be done in a concerted and coordinated manner for the patient to achieve the proper result. It is important to understand that anxiety, self-doubt and depression can also mitigate against the successful outcome in patients with FMS. When necessary, referral of an FMS patient with such symptoms to a counselor and possibly even to a psychiatrist would be a reasonable thing to do and can be very therapeutic. It is important to explain to the patient that even though he or she may need to see a mental health professional, the FMS is not a psychological problem; rather, they may need specific psychological/pyschiatric intervention in order to handle the stresses that this chronic condition imposes upon them and their loved ones.

The key to FMS treatment, in my opinion, is coordination of different modalities of care, individualization of treatment, education, support, and constant reassessment of the treatment modalities in order for the patient to get optimal care. This, of course, includes the identification and elimination/amelioration of perpetuating factors and the use of counseling where appropriate.

Medically reviewed and edited by Thomas J. Romano, M.D., Ph.D., FACP, FACR

Address: **Dr. Thomas J. Romano**
30 Medical Park, Suite 201
Wheeling, WV 26003
Phone: (304) 243-1760 • Fax (304) 243-1379

Taking Charge of Fibromyalgia Educational Program

We have developed a five to six hour educational class which coordinates with this patient handbook. The purpose of the class is to educate patients with fibromyalgia on the most up-to-date information on their condition, enabling them to become the primary movers in the management of their illness.

The class is designed so that it can be taught in a day-long seminar format, or it can be broken down into smaller segments of two to three hours over a period of time, according to your needs.

We have been teaching this class at Abbott-Northwestern Hospital in Minneapolis, Minnesota, six times a year since the fall of 1991, and in Toledo, Ohio, two to three times a year at Toledo Hospital since 1993. Other hospitals, rehabilitation centers, support groups and individuals have purchased the program to teach in their local area. The class is useful for newly diagnosed patients, their families, health care professionals and others needing information on fibromyalgia. It helps them gain a better understanding of this condition and facilitates an awareness in the community of fibromyalgia syndrome. CEU credits are available in Minnesota and Ohio and reciprocating states for various health care professionals.

The program includes a teaching manual, colored slides which correspond to the information in the patient handbook and a patient handbook. Handbooks are also available at a reduced price when purchased in quantity.

Ordering information can be found on our order form in the back of this book. You may look at samples of our colored slides on our website: fmsedsys.com. Please contact us personally if you have specific questions or would like us to teach a class in your area.

Julie Kelly, M.S., R.N.
(612) 473-6218

Rosalie Devonshire, M.S.W.
(201) 785-1128